Epilepsy, Behaviour and
Cognitive Function

Epilepsy, Behaviour and Cognitive Function

Stratford-upon-Avon Symposium
November 1987

Edited by

MICHAEL R. TRIMBLE
Consultant Physician in Psychological Medicine,
National Hospitals for Nervous Diseases,
and Raymond Way Senior Lecturer
in Behavioural Neurology, Institute
of Neurology, London

and

EDWARD H. REYNOLDS
Consultant Neurologist, Maudsley and King's
College Hospitals, London

A Wiley Medical Publication

JOHN WILEY & SONS
Chichester · New York · Brisbane · Toronto · Singapore

ISBN 0 471 91953 5

Typeset by Inforum Ltd, Portsmouth.
Printed and bound in Great Britain by Mackays of Chatham plc, Kent

Contents

Chairmen and Contributors.. vii
Acknowledgements viii
Preface ix

Section I

1 Historical aspects
   E.H. Reynolds 3
2 Methods and problems in the assessment of cognitive function in
   epileptic patients
   J. Ossetin 9
3 Methods and problems in the assessment of behaviour disorders
   in epileptic patients
   P.J. Thompson 27
Discussion 41

Section II

4 Seizures, EEG discharges and cognition
   C.D. Binnie 45
5 Seizures, EEG discharges and behaviour
   P.B.C. Fenwick 51
6 Anticonvulsants, seizures and performance: the Veteran's
   Administration experience
   D.B. Smith 67
Discussion 79

Section III

7   Educational needs and epilepsy in childhood
    E.M. Ross and P. Tookey 87
8   Cognitive function and behaviour in children
    C.A. Cull 97
9   Cognitive deterioration in children with epilepsy
    F.M.C. Besag 113
Discussion 129

Section IV

10 Anticonvulsant drugs: mood and cognitive function
    M.R. Trimble 135
11 Epilepsy and mood
    M.M. Robertson 145
Discussion 159

Section V

12 Memory and epilepsy
    P. Loiseau, E. Strube and J.-L. Signoret 165
13 Dementia in epileptic patients
    S.W. Brown and M. Vaughan 177
14 Late onset seizures and dementia: a review of epidemiology and
    aetiology
    S.D. Shorvon 189
Discussion 199

General discussion 201

Index 208

Chairmen and Contributors

F.M.C. Besag, *Lingfield Hospital School, Surrey, UK*
Colin D. Binnie, *The Maudsley Hospital, London, UK*
Stephen W. Brown, *The David Lewis Centre for Epilepsy, Warford, Cheshire, UK*
D.W. Chadwick, *Walton Hospital, Liverpool, UK*
J.A. Corbett, *Lea Castle Hospital, Kidderminster, UK*
Christine A. Cull, *The David Lewis Centre for Epilepsy, Warford, Cheshire, UK*
Peter B.C. Fenwick, *The Maudsley Hospital, London, UK*
Pierre Loiseau, *Clinique Neurologique, Hôpital Pellegrin, Université de Bordeaux II, France*
Jolanta Ossetin, *Institute of Psychiatry, London, UK*
E. H. Reynolds, *Maudsley and King's College Hospitals, London, UK*
Mary M. Robertson, *The Middlesex Hospital, London, UK*
Euan M. Ross, *Charing Cross Hospital and Institute of Child Health, London, UK*
Simon D. Shorvon, *National Hospitals for Nervous Diseases and Institute of Neurology, London, UK*
Jean-Louis Signoret, *Clinique des Maladies du Système Nerveux, Hôpital de la Salpêtrière, Université de Paris VI, France*
Dennis B. Smith, *Comprehensive Epilepsy Program of Oregon, Good Samaritan Hospital and Medical Center, Portland, Oregon, USA*
Evelyn Strube, *Clinique Neurologique, Hôpital Pellegrin, Université de Bordeaux II, France*
P.J. Thompson, *The Chalfont Centre for Epilepsy, Chalfont St Peter, Buckinghamshire, UK*
Pat Tookey, *Charing Cross Hospital and Institute of Child Health, London, UK*
Michael R. Trimble, *National Hospitals for Nervous Diseases and Institute of Neurology, London, UK*
Margaret Vaughan, *The David Lewis Centre for Epilepsy, Warford, Cheshire, UK*

Acknowledgements

The editors gratefully acknowledge the support of Ciba Geigy who helped coordinate the symposium on which this book was based. They are also deeply indebted to all the speakers for providing manuscripts for this book and for their vigorous participation in the meeting.

Preface

It has recently become clear that the majority of patients with epilepsy can have their seizures managed successfully. However, there remains a proportion of patients who fail to achieve adequate seizure control with modern anticonvulsant treatments using serum level monitoring and all of the advances of recent technology. Further, there are a significant number of patients, either with or without continuing seizures, who suffer from the neurological and psychosocial consequences of having epilepsy. Important amongst these are cognitive and behavioural complications, which have attracted a great deal of interest in recent years although few publications have been specifically orientated towards exploring these areas.

In order to produce this book, a symposium was organized at Stratford-upon-Avon in late 1987 at which a number of specialists in epilepsy who also have a specific interest in cognitive function and behaviour, were brought together. An invited audience also attended, and the final production represents papers catalysed by that meeting and some of the more interesting discussion. It is not intended that this should be a complete manual of cognitive and behavioural associations of epilepsy; that must wait for some future date. However, it is hoped that the book will be of interest to those who manage adults and children with epilepsy, and who are aware of the frequency with which the problems discussed here occur.

M.R. TRIMBLE
E.H. REYNOLDS

Section I

Epilepsy, Behaviour and Cognitive Function
Edited by M.R. Trimble and E.H. Reynolds
© 1988 John Wiley & Sons Ltd

1

Historical aspects

E.H. REYNOLDS
Maudsley and King's College Hospitals, London

Cassius: But soft, I pray you. What, did Caesar swoon?
Casca: He fell down in the market-place, and foam'd at mouth, and was speechless.
Brutus: 'Tis very like. He hath the falling sickness.
Cassius: No, Caesar hath it not; but you, and I,
And honest Casca, we have the falling sickness.

From
Julius Caesar, I,ii, by William Shakespeare.

The relationship between epilepsy and its behavioural or mental associations has always been a matter of great interest, debate and controversy. Before discussing current views on this contentious subject it is therefore appropriate to consider some of our ancestors' observations and opinions. There is an enormous historical legacy which has no doubt shaped our own, as well as public, attitudes to epilepsy. This has been reviewed in the classic work of Temkin (1945) which covers the period until the end of the nineteenth century. Other more recent contributions have been those of Lennox and Lennox (1960), Guerrant et al. (1962), Hill (1981) and Berrios (1984).

THE GRAECO-ROMAN PERIOD

The Greeks believed epilepsy to be a sacred disease, that is the result of the invasion of the body by a god. Only a god could deprive a healthy man of his senses, throw him to the ground, convulse him and then rapidly restore him to his former self again. The remarkable thing about Hippocrates' famous treatise on the 'Sacred Disease' was his opinion that epilepsy was *not* sacred, that the

Table 1.   Nineteenth century views of mental disorders associated with epilepsy

	Psychiatrists			Neurologists	
	N	% with mental disorder		N	% with mental disorder
Esquirol (1838)	385	80	Herpin (1852)	38	2.5
Morel (1857)	?	100	Reynolds (1861)	62	18
			Gowers (1881)	1085	7

human body could not be polluted by a god, and that the brain was the seat of this disease. He had to wait nearly 25 centuries for his hypothesis to be generally accepted!

The gods occupied heavenly spheres, one of which was the moon. Hence the word *lunatic* was first applied to sufferers of epilepsy. In contrast, mad people were *maniacs* whose madness was a result of invasion of the body by devils or evil spirits. However the distinction soon became blurred and epileptic patients were regarded as both lunatic and maniac. In the gospel account of St Mark (9, 17–27) it was a 'foul spirit' that was cast out of the young man with fits. What did Cassius mean when he said that he, Brutus and Casca (who were plotting to murder Caesar) had the falling sickness? That they were mad?

The association of epilepsy with mental disturbance persisted in the public mind right up to the nineteenth century.

THE NINETEENTH CENTURY

The process of distinguishing epilepsy from madness began in the nineteenth century and was linked with the development of neurology as a new and independent discipline. At the beginning and throughout most of the century epilepsy was still primarily the concern of alienists, the forerunners of modern psychiatrists, in charge of institutions such as the Salpêtrière, in France. The French alienists Morel and Esquirol were influential in perpetuating the view that most epileptic patients were mentally disturbed, and indeed Morel's famous 'degeneracy' theory was applied to the mentally ill with and without

Table 2.   Obscure or vague forms of epilepsy

Larval
Equivalent
Masked
Subictal
Subclinical

epilepsy. Epilepsy remained an integral part of psychiatric nosology. Such views were apparently accepted by English psychiatrists, including Maudsley.

It was the new neurologists who began to challenge these deeply entrenched concepts as they encountered much epilepsy without mental illness in their private practice. Table 1 contrasts the perspectives of Herpin (1852), Reynolds (1861) and Gowers (1881) with those of Esquirol (1838) and Morel (1857) on the association epilepsy and mental change. Even though Gowers is often quoted as stating that the mental state of the epileptic is frequently impaired, in fact he found that this was conspicuous in only 7% of his large series, slight degrees of memory impairment being discounted.

According to Berrios (1984), as the neurological perspective of epilepsy began to develop, the 'psychiatrists' invented a new strategy for keeping epilepsy in the psychiatric camp. New and obscure forms of epilepsy, such as 'larval' or 'masked' epilepsy or 'epileptic equivalent' were hypothesized to embrace vaguely paroxysmal forms of psychological disorder in the absence of any overt seizures. The French 'psychiatrists' Morel (1860) and Falret (1860) were again in the vanguard of this movement. This trend is still with us today, but following the discovery of the EEG by Berger newer words such as 'subclinical' and 'subictal' have replaced the earlier inventions (Table 2). Furthermore these concepts are advanced now not only by psychiatrists, but to some extent by neurologists and clinical neurophysiologists.

HUGHLINGS JACKSON

In the latter half of the nineteenth century views about epilepsy were radically changed by Jackson (1873) who suggested that the word should be redefined in *neurophysiological* rather than clinical terms, as follows:

> Epilepsy is the name for occasional, sudden, excessive, rapid and local discharges of grey matter.

This was the first neuronal theory of epilepsy, the foundation stone of our modern understanding of epilepsy. However, it brought with it certain complications. Like the psychiatrists with their 'masked' or 'larval' epilepsy, Jackson began to see epilepsy everywhere. This is illustrated for example in his statement that 'a sneeze is a sort of healthy epilepsy'. To his credit he recognized this problem, and in his Lumleian lectures (1890) reverted to an earlier *clinical* definition of epilepsy:

> I formerly used the term 'epilepsy' generically for all excessive discharges of the cortex and their consequences . . . I now use the term 'epilepsy' for that neurosis which is often called 'genuine' or 'ordinary' epilepsy, and for that only.

This semantic retreat by Jackson is apparently not well known and it was later overtaken by the discovery of the EEG. Although Berger himself did not understand English and possibly had never heard of Jackson, much less read his papers, a later generation of clinical neurophysiologists were convinced that the 'spikes' and other 'epileptiform' tracings that Berger and his successors had discovered corresponded with Jackson's intuitive neurophysiological definition of epilepsy (Reynolds, 1986).

One spin-off from Jackson's neurophysiological definition of epilepsy was that it was now possible to classify the mental manifestations of epilepsy into ictal and interictal, and later peri- or postictal. Jackson's own descriptions of 'dreamy states' represented an early attempt at defining ictal mental states.

THE TWENTIETH CENTURY

At the beginning of this century the psychiatrists' views about epilepsy still dominated the literature. Guerrant et al. (1962) describe three new phases of evolution of thinking since then. In the early part of this century the concept of the epileptic character held sway. According to this view the epileptic patient could be identified by his vulnerability to certain personality traits, mostly of an unfavourable or antisocial nature. Later, with the studies of Lennox in the 1930s and 1940s (see Lennox and Lennox, 1960), it became more widely accepted that most epileptic patients had normal mental states. This was really an extension of the observations first hinted at by the nineteenth-century neurologists (Table 1). The culmination of this process is that only in the last 30 years has the diagnosis 'epilepsy per se' finally been removed from national and international classifications of psychiatric illness (Hill, 1981).

Then the publication of a paper by Gibbs et al. (1948) ushered in what Guerrant et al. (1962) have called the era of 'psychomotor peculiarity'. In their electrophysiological study of patients with psychomotor seizures Gibbs et al. were impressed with the association of EEG abnormalities in the anterior temporal area and disturbances in personality. Since then the concept has expanded and an enormous and controversial literature has evolved relating temporal lobe epilepsy not only to personality disorder, but to aggression, schizophrenia-like psychoses, and much else. In many ways the personality debate is a rerun of the early twentieth-century controversy about epileptic character, but this time applied only to patients with a specific type of epilepsy!

The latter period of this century has been characterized by steadily increasing scientific study of the relationship between epilepsy and mental disturbance of all kinds. Epidemiological studies (Pond, 1981) have suggestd that as many as one-third or more patients with active epilepsy have significantly disabling additional psychological problems. They range in character from the cognitive impairment and behavioural disorders to be discussed in this book to psychiatric illness of all types, especially depression and anxiety. Instead of all-embracing 'degeneracy', 'personality' and 'temporal lobe' theories, recent research has begun to concentrate on the wide range of complex biological and psychosocial factors which exert their influence to varying degrees in children, adolescents or adults with epilepsy. These include the effects of: seizures of different types and combination; the duration and severity of the epilepsy; the age of onset of the disorder and the degree of maturation of the nervous system; the site of and degree of brain damage, whether pre- or postictal; the amount and duration of anti-epileptic therapy and its metabolic consequences; genetic factors; electroencephalographic abnormalities; neurophysiological mechanisms, such as kindling; and the influence of family, school, employment (or lack of it), and a whole range of environmental, social and psychodynamic factors. These studies have been assisted by new methods for quantitating psychometric performance, behaviour and psychopathology, and by new sophisticated techniques for clinical, electrophysiological and pharmacological monitoring and brain imaging. For example, when Trimble and Reynolds (1976) reviewed the literature on the mental effects of anti-epileptic drugs it was clear that there had been very little consideration, and much less adequate investigation, of this particular aspect. Now, just over a decade later, there has been a remarkable growth in interest and study of the subject (see chapters 6, 9, 10 and 11).

The nature, scale and complexity of its associated psychological disorders emphasize that epilepsy sits firmly on the bridge or interface between neurology and psychiatry and that the study of these associations can be expected to illuminate other aspects of these two disciplines (Reynolds and Trimble, 1981, 1989).

REFERENCES

BERRIOS, G.E. (1984) Epilepsy and insanity during the early 19th century. *Arch. Neurol.*, **41**, 978–981.

ESQUIROL, J.E.D. (1838) *Des Maladies Mentales*, J.B. Baillière, Paris.

FALRET, J. (1860–1861) De l'état mental des épileptiques, *Arch.Gen.Med.*, **16**, 661–679; **17**, 461–491; **18**, 423–443.

GIBBS, E.L., GIBBS, F.A., and FUSTER, B. (1948) Psychomotor epilepsy, *Arch.Neurol.*, **60**, 331–339.

GOWERS, W.R. (1881) *Epilepsy and Other Chronic Convulsive Disorders*. Churchill, London.

GUERRANT, J., ANDERSON, W.W., FISCHER, A., WEINSTEIN, M.R., JAROS, R.M. and DESKINS, A. (1962) *Personality in Epilepsy*. Thomas, Springfield, Ill.

HERPIN, T. (1852) *Du Prognostic et du Traitement Curatif de L'Epilepsie*. J.B. Baillière, Paris.

HILL, D. (1981) Historical review. In *Epilepsy and Psychiatry* (eds E.H. REYNOLDS and M.R. TRIMBLE), pp.1–11, Churchill Livingstone, Edinburgh.

JACKSON, J.H. (1873) On the anatomical, physiological, and pathological investigation of epilepsies. *Reports of the West Riding Lunatic Asylum*, **3**, 315–339.

JACKSON, J.H. (1890) On convulsive seizures. *Br.Med.J.*, **1**, 703–707.

LENNOX, W.G. and LENNOX, M.A. (1960) *Epilepsy and Related Disorders*. Little, Brown, Boston.

MOREL, B.A. (1857) *Traité des Dégénérescences Physiques, Intellectuelles et Morales de L'Espèce Humain et des Causes qui Produisent ses Variétés Maladaptives*, Vol. 1. Baillière, Paris.

MOREL, B.A. (1860) D'une forme de délire, suite d'une sur excitation nerveuse se rattachant a une variété non encore decrite d'épilepsie (épilepsie larvée). *Gaz.Hebdomad. Med.Chir.*, **7**, 773–775, 819–821, 836–841.

POND, D. (1981) Epidemiology of the psychiatric disorders of epilepsy. In *Epilepsy and Psychiatry* (eds E.H. REYNOLDS and M.R. TRIMBLE), pp.27–32, Churchill Livingstone, Edinburgh.

REYNOLDS, J.R. (1861) *Epilepsy; Its Symptoms, Treatment and Relation to Other Chronic Convulsive Disorders*. Churchill, London.

REYNOLDS, E.H. (1986) The clinical concept of epilepsy: an historical perspective. In *What is Epilepsy?* (eds M.R. TRIMBLE and E.H. REYNOLDS), pp. 1–7. Churchill Livingstone, Edinburgh.

REYNOLDS, E.H. and TRIMBLE, M.R. (eds) (1981) *Epilepsy and Psychiatry*. Churchill Livingstone, Edinburgh.

REYNOLDS, E.H. and TRIMBLE, M.R. (eds) (1989) *The Bridge between Neurology and Psychiatry*. Churchill Livingstone, Edinburgh.

TEMKIN, O. (1945) *The Falling Sickness*. The Johns Hopkins Press, Baltimore.

TRIMBLE, M.R. and REYNOLDS, E.H. (1976) Anticonvulsant drugs and mental symptoms: a review. *Psychological Medicine*, **6**, 169–178.

TRIMBLE, M.R. and REYNOLDS, E.H. (eds) (1986) *What is Epilepsy?* Churchill Livingstone, Edinburgh.

2

Methods and problems in the assessment of cognitive function in epileptic patients

JOLANTA OSSETIN
Institute of Psychiatry, London

INTRODUCTION

The concern over the mental functioning of patients with epilepsy has a long history (Chapter 1). Despite this, however, between 1950 and 1965 only 0.2% of 17,771 articles published on epilepsy included measures of intellectual functions (Penry, 1976). More recently, there has been a steady increase in the number of such studies because of a growing recognition of the importance of assessing intellectual functions for the diagnosis and prognosis of epileptic patients. It has also been appreciated that intellectual assessment plays an important part in the clinical management of epilepsy, so that a balance is kept between seizure control and the potentially adverse effects of antiepileptic drugs on mental functioning.

The methods used in assessing cognitive functions have undergone a considerable development from the early days, when the estimates were based solely on clinical impressions (e.g. Turner, 1907). The development of intelligence tests and neuropsychological test batteries, and the construction of memory tests and tests of specific cognitive functions, have given the clinicians and researchers a wide selection of tools. Furthermore, developments in the field of microcomputers have stimulated the construction of computer-based tests which can be efficiently administered and scored.

Many of the tests with epileptic patients have been borrowed and adapted from the research of experimental psychologists investigating general mechanisms of cognitive functions in normal and abnormal subjects. Many different workers have put forward different theories and models of cognitive functions and this has been associated with differences in the methods used in testing. The lack of agreement in the field of experimental cognitive psychology has been reflected in the clinical application of tests. Different clinicians and clinical research workers have selected the same tests to assess different cognitive functions and, conversely, a variety of tests have been used to assess purportedly the same function. On the whole, clinical research workers have put aside the theoretical issues and adopted an empirical approach, in which certain tests are selected, described, and the resulting measurements reported. The selection of tests has been guided by clinical observation, patients' complaints, and also the particular interests of a given medical and research centre.

The aim of this chapter is to examine some of the most frequently utilized tools in cognitive assessment of epileptic patients and to discuss the problems encountered in the interpretation of various studies. The assessment in three areas will be considered: intelligence, memory and specific cognitive functions. This review does not attempt to be exhaustive, but aims to select studies which help to highlight the problems associated with methodology.

ASSESSMENT OF INTELLIGENCE

Since the 1950s, the Wechsler scales, the WAIS and the WISC, have been the most commonly employed instruments for the assessment of intelligence in patients with epilepsy.

Level of intelligence

Since the early decades of this century the question has been asked whether the IQ of people with epilepsy was different from that of the normal population. Lower-than-normal IQ was found in epileptic patients with underlying brain damage (Yacorzynski and Arieff, 1942; Arieff and Yacorzynski, 1942), in patients with a relatively greater seizure frequency (Keith et al., 1955) and in institutionalized patients. A recent large-scale study of 622 epileptic adult out-patients has shown a normal WAIS scores distribution, though patients with secondarily generalized tonic-clonic seizures had significantly lower IQs (Smith et al., 1986). Children with epilepsy have been found to have a similar IQ to their non-epileptic siblings, although there was more variability in IQ and a higher rate of mental retardation among the patients. Both these differences disappeared when children who were impaired since infancy were excluded (Ellenberg et al., 1986).

There is a wide range of abilities among epileptic patients, which extends between mental retardation and very superior level of functioning. Therefore, attempts to answer a general question about intelligence level in epileptic populations are not well directed. More recently it has been accepted that several factors, such as type of seizure, age of onset, severity of epilepsy, brain damage, heredity and anticonvulsant drugs affect mental function in epileptic patients. Most of the studies have been carried out with heterogeneous groups of patients, and therefore the results are difficult to interpret.

An additional problem is that conclusions have been reached on the basis of a single assessment of the IQ of epileptic patients. The reliability, however, of the IQ measurement in the epileptic population is uncertain, because of marked fluctuations in retest scores already noted in early studies of Patterson and Fonner (1928) and Dawson and Conn (1929), and also reported in more recent investigations (e.g. Seidenberg et al., 1981; Smith et al., 1986).

Deterioration of intelligence

Studies have indicated that, in general, no deterioration of intelligence occurs in a majority of patients with epilepsy except for certain groups (see review by Lesser et al., 1986). Rodin (1968) found a slight but significant fall in Performance IQ for patients with initially high IQ, and those with high seizure frequency. Bourgeois et al. (1983) found no deterioration of IQ in a large group of children with epilepsy except in a small subgroup of patients. These patients had a higher incidence of toxic serum drug levels, earlier onset of seizures and poorer control of seizures. Control of seizures was found to be associated with IQ in a study by Rodin et al. (1986), who noted a stable or increased IQ for patients in remission, but a decrease in IQ for patients with poorly controlled epilepsy. These changes were small, however, and not statistically significant. There have been reports of a marked deterioration of IQ in over 15% of residential school patients (Corbett et al., 1985) and in patients with a history of status epilepticus or a considerable lifetime number of tonic-clonic seizures (Dodrill, 1986).

There are two major problems with assessing changes of intelligence over time. One is associated with the relative dependence of IQ scores on attained educational level. Dikmen (1980) found that among his patients, those with early onset epilepsy showed significant decreases on the WAIS, but he pointed out that these results could also be related to differences in years of schooling. The educational differences, in turn, could have either a cognitive or psychological basis. For example, Long and Moore (1979) found that parents of epileptic children have diminished expectations for their child's academic performance. The IQ deterioration might not therefore be linked causally to epilepsy, but to the psychosocial consequences of the disease.

The other problem stems from the practice effects of repeated IQ tests. Studies of recent outcome of the WAIS show a tendency for IQs to rise on the second testing, particularly for the Performance IQ, where the gains can be quite large (Matarazzo and Herman, 1984). Some reliability data on a single repeat WAIS administration for small groups of normal subjects and psychiatric and retarded patient are available, as well as tables for evaluating predicted retest changes in the WAIS scores (Knight and Shelton, 1983), but there are no data on reliability of multiple IQ administration. In addition, in epileptic patients the picture is compounded by the lack of means to distinguish between fluctuation improvement and practice effects. It needs to be noted, however, that Seidenberg et al. (1981) demonstrated that those patients whose seizure control improved showed increases in WAIS scores over and above what could be expected by the practice effects alone.

Lateralizing implication of Verbal-Performance IQ discrepancy

It is widely assumed that a differential performance on 'verbal' versus 'non-verbal' (Performance) tests on the WAIS reflect the lateralization of the lesion or focus of seizure discharge. Patients with a left hemisphere lesion or focus are expected to show a relative impairment on the Verbal IQ score while conversely, patients with right hemispheric lesion or focus will have impaired Performance IQ relative to their Verbal IQ (Reitan, 1955a; Kløve and Reitan, 1958; Black, 1974; also see a review by Guertin et al., 1966). For this reason the Wechsler scales have been used extensively in patients with temporal lobe epilepsy (TLE). The laterality effects of Wechsler scores in temporal lobe patients were found in some studies (Dennerll, 1964; Blakemore et al., 1966) but not in others. For example, Fedio and Mirsky (1969) found no Verbal–Performance IQ differences between groups of children with right TLE, left TLE, centrencephalic epilepsy and controls. More recently, Camfield et al. (1984) also failed to find laterality effects in the IQ scores of children with pure right versus pure left temporal lobe foci. It needs to be noted that the two latter studies have been carried out with children. The brain of a child has a greater plasticity, allowing for functional exchanges between the hemispheres (Smith and Sugar, 1975). On the whole, however, the evidence about lateralizing implications of the Wechsler scales is weak and not consistent for the following reasons. First, many so called 'non-verbal' tests require verbal–symbolic function for their solution, therefore impaired Performance IQ score may be due either to impaired left or right hemispheric function. Secondly, most of the Performance subtests are timed whilst Verbal tests are not. Any factor which affects the speed of mental processing, such as a lesion, irrespective of its location, EEG abnormality, or antiepileptic medication may result in a lower Performance than Verbal IQ score. Thirdly, according to Wechsler's own evidence, the relative balance between Verbal and Performance IQ depends on the overall intelligence level: as the Full Scale IQ decreases from 120 to 75 the proportion of subjects with higher Performance IQ than Verbal IQ increases from 21 to 74% (Wechsler, 1944).

Are the IQ tests necessary?

Besides using intelligence tests to assess a patient's general level of functioning, psychologists usually explore the pattern of subtests' scores for possible specific deficits. For example, poor performance on Digit Span suggests attentional disturbances, whilst the Digit Symbol test is sensitive to impairment with a lesion in any location (McFie, 1969). The Verbal–Performance discrepancy is a useful guide to lateralization in an individual case, but should be corroborated with relevant medical and educational data and other tests results (Bornstein, 1983).

The assessment of cognitive function of epileptic patients, whether for clinical or for research purposes, frequently includes several tests other than those of IQ. This results in very lengthy assessment sessions. Moehle et al. (1984) reported that a single assessment of their patients lasted between six and eight hours. In this, and similar studies, the reliability of the results may be threatened by the subjects' fatigue. In an attempt to reduce testing time, Kane et al. (1985) questioned whether the inclusion of the WAIS is necessary when neuropsychological test batteries, such as Halsted–Reitan or Luria–Nebraska are used. They found that although the WAIS had similar powers in the identification of brain damage to the batteries, each of the instruments showed differential sensitivity to various impairments despite some overlap between them. Similar findings were reported by Kupke and Lewis (1985) and they do not recommend that the WAIS be omitted from the assessments. But the use of shortened forms, consisting of four subtests (Similarities, Vocabulary, Picture Arrangement and Block Design), or only two subtests (Vocabulary and Block Design) has been suggested by Silverstein (1982). For research purposes, in order the match groups of subjects, this suggestion seems adequate.

Despite the problems associated with Wechsler scales, the IQ tests do appear to be useful, both for individual assessments, as well as in research studies. The intelligence tests on their own, however, are not sufficient to detect subtle changes of function, for which more specialized tests are required.

ASSESSMENT OF MEMORY AND LEARNING

Memory impairment associated with epilepsy was one of the earliest recognized deficits mentioned in the literature (Gowers, 1881). It is also the most common problem reported by the patients themselves.

Despite much concern expressed in the literature over the years, the studies evaluating memory function in epileptic patients are few, and most of those have not concentrated on it specifically, but have included some memory measures among other tests of cognitive functions. The dearth of studies of memory function in epileptic patients is evidenced by the yield of four Workshops on Memory Functions organized by the Swedish Branch of Epilepsy International and Ciba-Geigy between the years 1979 and 1985. Among the 57 published articles covering many topics often unrelated or remotely related to memory, only 14 have concentrated on memory in epileptic patients and only some of them reported measurement data. Only two authors have given attention to methodological problems. Stores (1981) has criticized the lack of agreement on what tests should be used to clarify the existence and nature of cognitive deficits. Nilsson (1980) has commented on memory testing, that 'there are almost just as many different methods as there are published studies', which makes integration of research difficult.

Methods of assessment of memory and learning

Memory assessments utilize several accepted divisions of memory function. Temporal division relates to Short-term Memory (STM), which is tested immediately after the presentation of material; and Long-term Memory (LTM), tested within an interval between 10 minutes and one hour. According to the type of material to be remembered, a distinction is drawn between verbal and non-verbal memory. Depending on the mode of testing two forms are used: recall, where the patient has to reproduce the material spontaneously and recognition, where the previously presented items have to be indicated from a larger array of similar items.

There are very few standardized memory tests. The most frequently used is the Wechsler Memory Scale (WMS; Wechsler, 1945), consisting of seven tests and yielding a Memory Quotient (MQ). In practice, a selection from the WMS is made and these are used independently. Verbal tests most commonly used are the Logical Memory (short prose passage), Associate Learning (learning of easy- and difficult-to-associate pairs of words) and Digit Span (the longest string of digits recalled). The only non-verbal test in WMS is Visual Reproduction (drawing geometrical designs of progressive difficulty level). Among other standardized memory tests are the Rey Auditory Verbal Learning Test (RAVLT; Rey, 1964) consisting of words recall on several successive trials, and the Benton Visual Retention Test (Benton, 1974), requiring reproduction of geometrical figures.

In addition, many non-standardized testing procedures have been used, such as word list recall and learning, and picture and face recognition. Some investigators used tasks relying heavily on fine sensory discrimination, for example, recognition of a token by its shade or texture (Scott et al., 1967) or recognition of perceptually degraded pictures of words or objects (Delaney et al., 1980). Other investigators used techniques derived from information-processing research; for instance, the Sternberg (1966) visual scanning task, which requires a rapid decision about the presence of absence of a probe digit in sequentially presented series of digits (MacLeod et al., 1978; Andrews et al., 1984). As can be seen from the above, there is a great variety of methods which appear to measure different aspects of memory. Some tests probe only the STM, like Digit Span from the WMS, some rely on intact sensory abilities, yet in others, such as the Sternberg task, unlike most memory tests, the principal measure is speed of response, the error assumed to be minimal.

In research with epileptic patients memory function has been assessed with respect to type of epilepsy (generalized versus focal) and types of impairment associated with right versus left seizure focus in temporal lobe epilepsy. The effects of EEG discharges and of anticonvulsant drugs on memory have also been investigated.

Memory function in patients with generalized versus focal epilepsy

Quadfasel and Pruyser (1955) compared patients with psychomotor and generalized seizures, who were matched for IQ, education, age of onset and duration of seizures. They used the WMS and found that patients with generalized seizures had normal memory function, but the patients with psychomotor seizures showed a verbal memory impairment. This deficit was associated with a general impairment in verbal functioning as measured by the verbal-conceptual tasks of the Wechsler–Bellevue. However, there were no differences between the groups on the Visual Reproduction test.

Consistent with the above results, Glowinski (1973) used the complete WMS and found that the temporal lobe group showed a significantly greater impairment than the centrencephalic group, particularly on the immediate recall of meaningful narrative (Logical Memory test). Language-related memory deficit in temporal lobe epilepsy was also found by Milberg et al. (1980). This conclusion was reached not by using a memory test, but by the results obtained on three WAIS subtests (Information, Vocabulary and Similarities), which were considered to be a measure of linguistic memory.

There are also reports of non-verbal memory deficits in patients with psychomotor seizures, particularly when combined with grand mal seizures. For example, Schwartz and Dennerll (1969) found such patients impaired on the immediate visual recall of the Bender–Gestalt test.

In contrast with the above studies, Loiseau et al. (1983) found that the TLE patients' memory function did not differ from controls, but the patients with primary generalized epilepsy showed memory impairment. But only two WMS tests were used, Digit Span and Visual Reproduction, and the RAVLT, which was modified; and the selection of tests may have influenced the results.

Memory function in right TLE versus left TLE patients

A number of studies have suggested that the side of lesion determines the kind of material more susceptible to deficit. Left-sided lesions result in memory impairment for verbal material, whilst right-sided for non-verbal material. The evidence for this pattern of deficits was obtained from surgical patients who had undergone a unilateral temporal lobectomy for treatment of epilepsy (e.g. Milner, 1965, 1970). But in patients without gross cerebral damage the evidence of interhemispheric differences for verbal and non-verbal material is less clear. For example, Quadfasel and Pruyser (1955) found that the verbal memory deficit in patients with psychomotor seizures was not related to lateralization of EEG focus. However, only six patients in the sample had a consistent unilateral spike discharge, and only one had a focus in the right hemisphere. Glowinski (1973) found no significant relationship between laterality of lesion and impairment of verbal and non-verbal memory, though in individual cases the deficit was in the predicted direction. More recently, both Loiseau et al. (1983) and Mungas et al. (1985) failed to find differences between the right- and left-TLE patients on the verbal memory test and the RAVLT.

Several studies distinguished between the STM and LTM impairment, or interpreted their results in terms of differential sensitivity on short- or long-term memory testing to deficits.

Ladavas et al. (1979) investigated left versus right hemisphere memory function as assessed by the STM and LTM performance on a variety of verbal and non-verbal tests. Although the STM tasks did not differentiate between the left and right temporal lobe foci patients, the LTM tasks did so, in the expected verbal/non-verbal direction. Similar results were obtained by Delaney et al. (1980) who found that differences between the right and left TLE patients were not apparent on immediate recall of either the verbal or non-verbal material, but only on delayed recall. The authors also noted that a recognition test or a test of perceptually degraded material did not disclose memory impairment, but free recall did.

Both the Ladavas et al. (1979) and Delaney et al. (1980) studies give rise to important methodological issues with respect to adequacy and power of memory tests. Positive or negative findings in studies may result equally from the actual presence or absence of an impairment, as from the failure of a particular test to reveal it. The danger of spurious results is greater in studies where experimental, non-standardized tests are used.

Subictal EEG discharges and memory function

Several investigators have pointed to the disruptive effects of subictal (subclinical) discharges on memory. Glowinski (1973) first proposed this as a 'tentative hypothesis', which was supported later by studies comparing memory performance with EEG recordings. For example, Loiseau et al. (1983) found that the patients with interictal bilateral spike and wave complexes had the poorest results on memory tests. Binnie and colleagues (Aarts et al., 1984; Binnie, see Chapter 4) have devised two computer-based verbal and non-verbal memory tasks which were performed by patients over an extended period (30–60 min) with simultaneous EEG and video monitoring. They observed an impairment on both tasks during spike or spike-wave discharges. A significant association was found between the locus of discharges and impairment on verbal and non-verbal tasks, which were affected by left and right discharges respectively. Discharges during stimulus presentation, but not during the response phase, were most disruptive of performance, which points to dependence of memory function on attention and vigilance. In fact most studies dealing with the effects of subictal discharges on cognition concentrated on these functions, rather than on memory, and will be discussed later.

Memory function and anticonvulsant drugs

In the last decade or so there has been an increasing awareness of the toxic effect of anticonvulsant drugs on cognitive function (e.g. Reynolds, 1975; Trimble and Reynolds, 1976) and particularly of the harmful effects of polytherapy (Reynolds and Shorvon, 1981). This may occur even when drugs are kept within the 'therapeutic range', but the studies which have dealt specifically with memory impairment and anticonvulsants are few.

MacLeod et al. (1978) investigated memory function in epileptic patients treated with medium and high therapeutic doses of phenobarbitone. They found impaired STM performance as measured by the Sternberg scanning task when the drug level was high. Access to LTM, as measured by a test of identifying letters as the same either by their appearance (e.g. 'AA') or their name (e.g. 'Aa'), was not affected.

The Sternberg task was also used by Andrewes et al. (1984, 1986), and revealed a relative memory impairment in patients treated with phenytoin, compared to those treated with carbamazepine. The Sternberg task and letter-identifying task (MacLeod et al., 1978) utilize time of response as a memory measure, have fast speeds of presentation and are carried out over a longer passage of time than most memory tests. It is arguable whether they are tests of memory, reaction time, or vigilance.

Thompson and Trimble (see Chapter 10) have investigated memory among other cognitive functions in a number of studies with epileptic patients, and volunteers given anti-epileptic drugs. They have consistently employed the same battery of tests. Their memory test consists of immediate and delayed recall of twenty words and twenty pictures, followed by a recognition test of the items embedded in distractor items. Thompson and Trimble (1982) found improved memory function in patients undergoing reduction in polytherapy or substitution of one of their drugs by carbamazepine. However, the number of patients in their study was small, eight different drugs were represented, and not all memory measures showed changes. In a study comparing cognitive functioning with high and lower serum levels of anticonvulsants, Thompson and Trimble (1983) found impaired memory on immediate recall when the levels of drugs were high, but no effect was seen on a delayed recall or recognition test. Among a series of studies evaluating cognitive effects of major anticonvulsants in normal volunteers, Thompson et al. (1981) found memory impairment on administration of phenytoin. A limitation of volunteer studies is that the short-term administration of a drug is not comparable to long-term treatment of patients, because cognitive effects may be either exacerbated or attentuated in long-term treatment. The possible problem is the potentially different effects of drugs on a normal brain compared with that of a patient with epilepsy.

ASSESSMENT OF OTHER SPECIFIC COGNITIVE FUNCTIONS

While global intellectual ability may be unaffected in a majority of patients with epilepsy, specific cognitive functions, such as mental speed, attention and vigilance may show subtle impairments, and therefore measures of these abilities are often included in assessment procedures.

The main interest has concentrated on the effects of EEG discharges and of anticonvulsant drugs on cognitive processing. But to date no specific pattern of cognitive dysfunction, either associated with seizure activity or with drug effects, has been established. This may be due to the multiple factors influencing cognitive functioning of epileptic patients, but also due to a wide variety of tests used in assessments.

Mental speed

Mental speed, or psychomotor speed, is most commonly measured by Reaction Time (RT). Simple Reaction Time (SRT) requires a response to a simple, unambiguous stimulus delivered at irregular intervals over a period of time. In Choice Reaction Time (CRT) alternative responses need to be made to two or more stimuli. There are differences of opinion whether the SRT or CRT is more sensitive to impairment (see review by Elsass, 1986), but some authors believe that the CRT is a better measure (e.g. Miller, 1970).

Schwab (1939) was the first who explored the effects of generalized spike-wave discharge on patients' performance using a Reaction Time test and simultaneous EEG recording. He found that during discharges there was a slowing of RT or no response was made. Hutt and Fairweather (1975) and Hutt et al. (1977) showed, however, that the characteristics of the RT task were important in revealing the impairment. When the rate of presentation was fast or slow no deficit was seen. On the other hand, impairment was revealed with an intermediate rate of presentation. Also, the more complex tasks were more susceptible to disturbance by the spike-wave bursts.

The effects of anticonvulsant drugs on mental speed have been investigated by several workers. Andrewes et al. (1984, 1986) compared performance of patients treated by monotherapy with CBZ or DPH and found that the SRT test and two CRT tests did not differentiate between the groups, although the CBZ group performed better on a test of perceptuo-motor coordination. Smith et al. (1986; Chapter 6) compared the performance of epileptic patients before and after one month of drug therapy, using a 'Discriminative Reaction Time' test. This test required the patient to reach the keys by moving the hand from a midline position to the right or left, depending on stimulus colour. The test revealed slowing of responses following initiation of drug treatment, but due to a much larger motor element in this test than in similar RT tasks in other studies, this could have been due to the motor slowing alone. In addition, in this large-scale study (n=622) no separate analysis for the individual drugs was reported, although there is evidence that their effects differ. For example, in a series of studies with volunteers, Thompson and Trimble observed that sodium valproate and clobazam caused slowing down of mental processing, particularly when task demands increased (Thompson and Trimble 1981a, b), while changes associated with carbamazepine occurred in relation to motor, rather than mental speed (Trimble and Thompson, 1983).

The results obtained by this team are difficult to compare with the findings of other authors, because their methodology of measuring mental speed is very different. They divide it into measures of perceptual speed, where a masking paradigm is used, and decision-making. In the masking task, the measure is the minimal time of display for a picture or a word or an object to be recognized. The decision-making task requires a verbal response about the colour of an object or its membership in a category. The measurement of speed of response in this task is obviously very different from the majority of tasks assessing mental speed, which require usually pressing a key or button. To assess motor speed, Thompson and Trimble used tapping rate between two metal plates with the dominant hand, non-dominant hand, and both hands simultaneously. They showed that reduction of polytherapy or substitution of one of the drugs by CBZ resulted in improved performance on this task, as well as on mental speed, measured as described above (Thompson and Trimble, 1982). There appears to be an inconsistency with respect to CBZ effects on motor function between this study in patients and the study with volunteers (Trimble and Thompson, 1983) which showed motor slowing on CBZ. This contradiction may be partly due to the limitations associated with the use of volunteers (which have been mentioned before), and partly to problems associated with evaluating the effects of individual drugs when patients are on polytherapy (Thompson and Trimble, 1982).

Attention, concentration and vigilance

Specific cognitive functions such as attention, concentration and vigilance are poorly defined in the studies, and the terms are frequently used interchangeably. The term vigilance refers to general reactivity of the organism to incoming stimuli, whilst attention implies more selective response to a given stimulus or stimuli, and presupposes at least a moderate level of vigilance (Bruhn, 1970). Most investigators however, do not make a clear distinction between attention, concentration and vigilance.

The most commonly used task in the assessment of vigilance or sustained attention is the Continuous Performance Test (CPT; Rosvold et al., 1956). In this test a series of letters of the alphabet is presented visually at the rate of one letter per second. The subject has to press a key whenever he notices a particular letter or a sequence of two letters, and he performs this task for a period of 10–20 minutes. Many versions of the CPT have been employed in studies, using visual or auditory stimuli, different rates of stimulus presentation, and different length of tests. These procedural details have often not been sufficiently described in the reports.

Impairment of sustained attention, as measured by the CPT, in patients with centrencephalic epilepsy was already noted in early studies (Mirsky et al., 1960; Lansdell and Mirsky, 1964). Mirsky and Van Buren (1965) have demonstrated that this deficit was associated with spike-wave activity, as shown by simultaneous EEG monitoring and task performance. Symmetrical, regular and synchronous bursts produced more deficit in performance than other bursts. But the effects were not consistent, as some patients showed impaired attention in the absence of bursts whilst others showed no change in performance during the bursts. One of the reasons for this may lie in the differential effects of bursts depending on their duration, as shown by Goode et al. (1970). In this study there was a high incidence of errors with bursts longer than 3 s, whilst shorter paroxysms had no effects on performance. The above studies point to the importance of carrying out psychological testing of patients in conjunction with the EEG recording.

There have been reports of inattentiveness of children with epilepsy (e.g. Whitmore and Holdsworth, 1971; Stores, 1973), but the outcome of the studies is not clear. For instance, Stores et al. (1978) found impaired attention in epileptic boys but not girls. In this study the CPT was used and the differences emerged in the second 8 min of the tests. In most other studies the statistical analysis of the data was not detailed enough to reflect changes of performance over time.

Another test which has been used in the assessment of attention or concentration is the visual or auditory scanning task. In this test, the patient is required to cross out one designated letter or number from a page with randomized letters or numbers. In the auditory version the stimuli are delivered through earphones and the response may be made by pressing a key. The Stroop test has also been used by investigators. It requires naming of the colour in which a word is written, the word being a name of a colour, but the colour and word are incongruent. For example, for the word 'red' written in green ink the correct answer is 'green'. Concentration is required to suppress a more 'natural' response of reading the word as written.

Both the Stroop test and the visual scanning task have been used in a series of drug studies of Thompson and Trimble. For example, in the study of patients with high or low anticonvulsant serum levels (Thompson and Trimble, 1983), a deficit in concentration was observed in the high drug level condition. But this deficit was only seen on the performance of the visual scanning task when it was presented in conjunction with auditory distraction. The Stroop test was performed somewhat faster and more accurately by the patients with a higher drug level. The number of subjects in the study was small and five major anticonvulsants were considered jointly, thus the results are difficult to interpret. In the study of the effects of reduction of polytherapy or substituting one of the drugs with CBZ (Thompson and Trimble, 1982) the performance on the visual scanning task improved in patients after changes in therapy, but the Stroop test showed no significant changes. These results illustrate the difficulties of interpretation when only some of the selected measures of a given function show change or when the measures yield contradictory results. The reasons for this may lie equally in the patients' characteristics, for example, different level of intelligence, different drug regimen, etc. as in different characteristics of tests used to measure the same function.

CONCLUDING REMARKS

The assessment of intelligence of patients with epilepsy does not pose many methodological problems from the point of view of the instruments used. Also all investigators have used Wechsler scales which are well standardized, well established, and their properties much researched. Thus the comparability across the studies may be limited by other factors, such as the unrepresentative nature of a studied group of patients for the wider population of patients with epilepsy, the heterogeneity of the patient groups, and the size of groups under investigation. These problems could be overcome by undertaking multicentre studies, where large numbers and careful grouping of patients could be assured. The methodological problem of the fluctuating IQ scores of epileptic patients could also be partially overcome by large numbers under study. The problem of practice effects on repeated IQ administration in prospective studies can be helped by careful spacing of the assessments. Including groups of normal controls tested at the same time intervals would also be very useful.

Assessment of memory and specific cognitive functions poses more serious problems. Although deficits in these abilities among patients with epilepsy are widely believed, the database is poor. There is a great variety of methods of assessment and almost every investigator has used different tests. The tests differ with respect to sensory modality, speed of presentation, duration of task, and type of response. As even small procedural changes in the same test may lead to different results, it is not surprising that the outcome of studies has not been consistent, and comparisons between the studies are difficult.

The theoretical underpinning of many tests is poor, or tests are chosen which are built on a narrow model of doubtful clinical significance such as, for example, the Sternberg memory scanning task. There is a lack of working definitions of basic terms and confusion in terminology, particularly in relation to specific cognitive functions, where such terms as attention, concentration and vigilance are used interchangeably.

Most of the tests of memory and specific cognitive functions have not been standardized, and those which have, have poor normative data. The tests have no age-related data, though many cognitive abilities show developmental changes. For example, children have longer reaction times than adults (Anderson et al., 1984). Although some investigators reported that they had used tests free of practice effects, the data on repeated test administration have not been presented. There are also other problems with interpretation of results. Many of the tests yield two measures – time and error – but there are no statistical methods to combine them into a summary score. As there is a trade-off between speed and accuracy, it is difficult to decide whether a patient has improved or deteriorated when these two scores point in opposite directions, on repeat of the test. Where several measures of the same function have been used in a study, or one test yielded several scores, over-generalized conclusions of impairment have been reached when only one of the scores showed decrement. So far no question has been raised over the possibility that scores in tests of memory and specific cognitive functions may be subject to fluctuations in performance, perhaps even to a greater degree than is the case with the IQ tests.

From many studies it has transpired that most cognitive tasks are composed of at least three phases: sensory input, integration or decision and response. Investigators have pointed out that sometimes deficits may occur in only one of these phases. This observation needs to be followed up by refining the existing tests through task analysis. Trying out one task at a time, and varying systematically only one of its parameters in turn, such as rate of presentation or level of difficulty of decision, should reveal the potential sources of decrement in performance and the type of tasks that are sensitive to this decrement. For this purpose single case-studies are eminently suitable. On the other hand, conceptual clarification and agreement on a basic set of methods of assessment of memory and specific cognitive functions is necessary. The use of the same tests combined with collaborative effort of various centres, would allow for homogeneous grouping of patients and more conclusive findings regarding the existence and nature of cognitive impairments in people with epilepsy.

REFERENCES

AARTS, J.H.P., BINNIE, C.D., SMIT, A.M. and WILKINS, A.J. (1984) Selective cognitive impairment during focal and generalized epileptiform EEG activity. *Brain*, **107**, 291–308.

ANDERSEN, K., STARCK, L., ROSÉN, I. and SVENSSON, E. (1984) The development of simple acoustic, reaction time in normal children. *Develop.Med.Child Neurol.*, **26**, 490–494.

ANDREWES, D.G., BULLEN, J.G., TOMLINSON, L., ELWES, R.D.C. and REYNOLDS, E.H. (1986) A comparative study of the cognitive effects of phenytoin and carbamazepine in new referrals with epilepsy. *Epilepsia*, **27**, 128–134.

ANDREWES, D.G., TOMLINSON, L., ELWES, R.D.C. and REYNOLDS, E.H. (1984) The influence of carbamazepine and phenytoin on memory and other aspects of cognitive function in new referrals with epilepsy, *Acta Neurol.Scand.*, **69**, 23–30.

ARIEFF, A.J. and YACORZYNSKI, G.K. (1942) Deterioration of patients with organic epilepsy. *J.Nerv.Ment.Dis.*, **96**, 49–55.

BENTON, A.L. (1974) *Revised Visual Retention Test: Manual.* Psychological Corporation, New York.

BINET, A. and SIMON, TH. (1905). Méthodes nouvelles pour le diagnostic du niveau intellectuel des anormaux. *Ann.Psychol.*, **11**, 191–244.

BLACK, F.W. (1974). Cognitive effects of unilateral brain lesions secondary to penetrating missile wounds. *Percept. Motor Skills*, **38**, 387–391.

BLAKEMORE, C.B., ETTLINGER, G. and FALCONER, M.A. (1966) Cognitive abilities in relation to the frequency of seizures and neuropathology of the temporal lobes in man. *J.Neurol.Neurosurg.Psychiat.*, **29**, 268–272.

BORNSTEIN, R.A. (1983). Verbal IQ–Performance IQ discrepancies on the Wechsler Adult Intelligence Scale–Revised in patients with unilateral or Bilateral Cerebral Dysfunction. *J.Consult.Clin.Psychol.*, **51**, 5, 779–780.

BOURGEOIS, B.F.D., PRENSKY, A.L., PALKES, H.S., TALENT, B.K. and BUSCH, S.G. (1983) Intelligence in epilepsy: a prospective study in children. *Ann.Neurol.*, **14**, 438–444.

BRUHN, P. (1970) Disturbance of vigilance in subcortical epilepsy. *Acta Neurol.Scand.*, **46**, 442–454.

CAMFIELD, P.R., GATES, R., RONEN, G., CAMFIELD, C., FERGUSON, A. and MACDONALD, G.W. (1984) Comparison of cognitive ability, personality profile, and school success in epileptic children with pure right versus left temporal lobe EEG foci. *Ann.Neurol.*, **15**, 122–126.

CORBETT, J.A., TRIMBLE, M.R. and NICOL, T.C. (1985) Behavioural and cognitive impairments in children with epilepsy: The long term effects of anticonvulsant therapy. *J.Am.Acad.Child Psychiatry*, **24**, 17–23.

DAWSON, S. and CONN, J. (1929). The intelligence of epileptic children. *Arch.Dis. Child.*, **4**, 142–151.

DELANEY, R.C., ROSEN, R.J., MATTSON, R.H. and NOVELLY, R.A. (1980) Memory function in focal epilepsy. A comparison of non-surgical unilateral temporal lobe and frontal lobe samples. *Cortex*, **16**, 103–117.

DENNERLL, R.D. (1964) Cognitive deficits and lateral brain dysfunction in temporal lobe epilepsy. *Epilepsia*, **5**, 177–191.

DIKMEN, S. (1980) Neuropsychological aspects of epilepsy. In *A Multidisciplinary Handbook of Epilepsy* (ed. B.P. HERMAN). Charles C. Thomas, Springfield, Illinois.

DODRILL, C.B. (1986) Correlates of generalized tonic-clonic seizures with intellectual, neuropsychological, emotional, and social function in patients with epilepsy. *Epilepsia*, **27**, 399–411.

ELLENBERG, J.H., HIRTZ, D.G. and NELSON, K.B. (1986) Do seizures in children cause intellectual deterioration? *N.Engl.J.Med.*, **314**, 1085–1088.

ELSASS, P. (1986) Continuous reaction times in cerebral dysfunction. *Acta Neurol. Scand.*, **73**, 225–246.

FEDIO, P. and MIRSKY, A.F. (1969) Selective intellectual deficits in children with temporal lobe or centrencephalic epilepsy. *Neuropsychologia*, **7**, 287–300.

GLOWINSKI, H. (1973) Cognitive deficits in temporal lobe epilepsy. An investigation of memory function. *J.Nerv.Ment.Dis.*, **137**, 129–137.

GOODE, D.J. PENRY, J.K. and DREIFUSS, F.E. (1970). Effects of paroxysmal spike-wave on continuous visual-motor performance. *Epilepsia*, **11**, 241–254.

GOWERS, W.R. (1881) *Epilepsy and Other Chronic Convulsive Diseases*. Churchill, London.

GUERTIN, W.H., LADD, C.E., FRANK, G.H., RABBIN, A.I. and HEISTER, D.S. (1966) Research with the Wechsler Intelligence Scales for Adults. *Psychol.Bull.*, **66**, 385–409.

HUTT, S.J. and FAIRWEATHER, H. (1975) Information processing during two types of EEG activity. *Electroenceph.Clin.Neurophysiol.*, **39**, 43–51.

HUTT, S.J., JACKSON, R.M., BELSHAM, A. and HIGGINS, G. (1968). Perceptual-motor behaviour in relation to blood phenobarbitone level: A preliminary report. *Dev.Med. Child Neurol.*, **10**, 626–632.

HUTT, S.J., NEWTON, J. and FAIRWEATHER, H. (1977) Choice reaction time and EEG activity, in children with epilepsy. *Neuropsychologia*, **15**, 257–267.

KANE, R.L., PARSONS, O.A. and GOLDSTEIN, G. (1985) Statistical relationships and discriminative accuracy of the Halsted-Reitan, Luria-Nebraska, and Wechsler IQ scores in the identification of brain damage. *J.Clin.Exp.Neuropsychol.*, **7**, 211–223.

KEITH, H.M., EWERT, J.C., GREEN, M.W. and GAGE, R.P. (1955) Mental status of children with convulsive disorders. *Neurol. (Minneapolis)*, **5**, 419–425.

KLØVE, H. and REITAN, R.M. (1958) The effects of dysphasia and spatial distortion on Wechsler-Bellevue results. *Arch.Neurol.Psychiat.*, **80**, 708–713.

KNIGHT, R.G. and SHELTON, E.J. (1983) Tables for evaluating predicted retest changes in Wechsler Adult Intelligence Scale Scores. *B.J.Clin.Psychol.*, **22**, 77–81.

KUPKE, T. and LEWIS, R. (1985) WAIS and neuropsychological tests: common and unique variance within an epileptic population. *J.Clin.Exp.Neuropsychol.*, **7**, 353–366.

LADAVAS, E., UMILTA, C. and PROVINCIALI, L. (1979) Hemisphere–dependent cognitive performances in epileptic patients. *Epilepsia*, **20**, 493–502.

LANSDELL, H. and MIRSKY, A.F. (1964) Attention in focal and centrencephalic epilepsy. *Exp.Neurol.*, **9**, 463–469.

LESSER, R.P., LUDERS, H., WYLLIE, E., DINNER, D.S. and MORRIS, H.H. (1986) Mental deterioration in epilepsy. *Epilepsia*, **27** (Suppl.2), S105–S123.

LOISEAU, P., STRUBE, E., BROUSTET, D., BATTELLOCHI, S., GOMENI, C. and MORSELLI, P.L. (1983) Learning impairment in epileptic patients. *Epilepsia*, **24**, 183–192.

LONG, C.G. and MOORE, J.R. (1979). Parental expectations for their epileptic children. *J.Child.Psychol.Psychiat.*, **20**, 299–312.

MACLEOD, C.M., DEKABAN, A.S. and HUNT, E. (1978) Memory impairment in epileptic patients: selective effects of phenobarbital concentration. *Science*, **202**, 1102–1104.

MATARAZZO, J.D. and HERMAN, D.O. (1984) Base rate data for the WAIS-R: Test–retest, stability and VIQ–PIQ differences. *J.Clin.Neuropyschol.*, **6**, 351–366.

McFIE, J. (1969) The diagnostic significance of disorders of higher nervous activity. In

Handbook of Clinical Neurology (eds P.J. VINKEN and G.W. BRUYN), Vol.4. ch.1. North-Holland, Amsterdam.

MILBERG, W., GREIFFENSTEIN, M., LEWIS, R. and ROURKE, D. (1980) Differentiation of temporal lobe and generalized seizure patients with the WAIS. *J.Consul.Clin. Psychol.*, **48**, 39–42.

MILLER, E. (1970) Simple and choice reaction time following severe head injury. *Cortex*, **6**, 121–127.

MILNER, B. (1965) Visually-guided maze learning in man: effects of bilateral hippocampal, bilateral frontal, and unilateral cerebral lesions. *Neuropsychologia*, **3**, 317–338.

MILNER, B. (1970) Memory and the medial temporal regions of the brain. In *Biology of Memory* (eds K.H. PRIBRAM and D.E. BROADBENT). Academic Press, New York.

MIRSKY, A.F. and VAN BUREN, J.M. (1965) On the nature of the 'absence' in centrencephalic epilepsy: A study of some behavioural, electroencephalographic and autonomic factors. *Electrocencephal.Clin.Neurophysiol.*, **18**, 334–348.

MIRSKY, A.F., PRIMAC, D.W., AJMONE MARSAN, C., ROSVOLD, H.E. and STEVENS, J.R. (1960) A comparison of the psychological test performance of patients with focal and nonfocal epilepsy. *Exp.Neurol.*, **2**, 75–89.

MOEHLE, K.A., BOLTER, J.F. and LONG, C.J. (1984) The relationship between neuropsychological functioning and psychopathology in temporal lobe epileptic patients. *Epilepsia*, **25**, 418–422.

MUNGAS, D., EHLERS, C., WALTON, N. and McCUTCHEN, B. (1985) Verbal learning differences in epileptic patients with left and right temporal lobe foci. *Epilepsia*, **26**, 340–345.

NILSSON, L.G. (1980) Methodological and theoretical considerations as a basis for an integration of research on memory functions in epileptic patients. *Acta Neurol. Scand.*, Suppl.80, 62, 62–74.

PATTERSON, H.A. and FONNER, D. (1928) Some observations on the intelligence quotient in epileptics. *Psychiat.Quart.*, **31**, 542–548.

PENRY, J.F. (1976) *Epilepsy Bibliography 1950–1975*, J.F. PENRY (ed.). Department of Health, Education and Welfare, Bethesda.

QUADFASEL, A.F. and PRUYSER, P.W. (1955) Cognitive deficits in patients with psychomotor epilepsy. *Epilepsia*, **4**, 80–90.

REITAN, R.M. (1955) Certain differential effects of left and right cerebral lesions in human adults. *J.Comparat.Physiol.Psychol.*, **48**, 474–477.

REY, A. (1964) '*L'Examen Clinique en Psychologie*. Presses Universitaires de France, Paris.

REYNOLDS, E.H. (1975). Chronic antiepileptic toxicity: A review. *Epilepsia*, **16**, 319–352.

REYNOLDS, E.H. and SHORVON, S.D. (1981) Monotherapy or polytherapy for epilepsy? *Epilepsia*, **22**, 1–10.

RODIN, E.A. (1968) *The Prognosis of Patients with Epilepsy*. C. Thomas, Springfield, Illinois.

RODIN, E., SCHMALTZ, S. and TUITLY, G. (1986) Intellectual functions of patients with childhood-onset epilepsy. *Dev.Med.Child Neurol.*, **28**, 25–33.

ROSVOLD, H.E., MIRSKY, A.F., SARASON, I., BRANSOME, E.D. and BECK, L.H. (1956) A continuous performance test for brain damage. *J.Consult.Psychol.*, **20**, 343–350.

SCHWAB, R.S. (1939) Method of measuring consciousness in attacks of petit mal epilepsy. *Arch.Neurol.Psychiat.*, **41**, 215–217.

SCHWARTZ, M.L. and DENNERLL, R.D., (1969) Immediate visual memory as a function of epileptic seizure type. *Cortex*, **5**, 69–74.

SCOTT, D.F., MOFFETT, A., MATHEWS, A. and ETTLINGER, G. (1967) The effect of epileptic discharges on learning and memory in patients. *Epilepsia*, **8**, 188–194.

SEIDENBERG, M., O'LEARY, D.S., BERENT, S. and BOLL, T. (1981). Changes in seizure frequency and test-retest scores on the Wechsler Adult Intelligence Scale. *Epilepsia*, **22**, 75–83.

SILVERSTEIN, A.B. (1982) Two- and four-subtest short forms of the Wechsler Adult Intelligence Scale – Revised. *J.Consult.Clin.Psych.*, **50**, 415–418.

SMITH, A. and SUGAR, O. (1975) Development of above normal language and intelligence 21 years after left hemispherectomy. *Neurology*, **25**, 813–818.

SMITH, D.B., CRAFT, B.R., COLLINS, J., MATTSON, R.H., CRAMER, J.A. and the VA Co-operative Study Group 118 (1986) Behavioural characteristics of epilepsy patients compared with normal controls. *Epilepsia*, **27**, 760–768.

STERNBERG, S. (1966) High speed scanning in human memory. *Science*, **153**, 652–654.

STORES, G. (1973) Studies of attention and seizure disorders. *Dev.Med.Child Neurol.*, **15**, 376–382.

STORES, G. (1981) Memory impairment in children with epilepsy. *Acta Neurol.Scand.*, Suppl. **89**, **64**, 21–27.

STORES, G., HART, J. and PIRAN, N. (1978) Inattentiveness in schoolchildren with epilepsy. *Epilepsia*, **19**, 169–175.

THOMPSON, P., HUPPERT, F.A. and TRIMBLE, M. (1981) Phenytoin and cognitive function: effects on normal volunteers and implications for epilepsy. *Br.J.Clin. Psychol.*, **20**, 155–162.

THOMPSON, P.J. and TRIMBLE, M.R. (1981a) Sodium valproate and cognitive functioning in normal volunteers. *Br.J.Clin.Pharmacol.*, **12**, 819–824.

THOMPSON, P.J. and TRIMBLE, M.R. (1981b) Clobazam and cognitive functions: effects in healthy volunteers. In *Clobazam: RSM International Congress and Symposium Series no. 43*, pp. 33–38, Academic Press, London.

THOMPSON, P.J. and TRIMBLE, M.R. (1982) Anticonvulsant drugs and cognitive functions. *Epilepsia*, **23**, 531–544.

THOMPSON, P.J. and TRIMBLE, M.R. (1983) Anticonvulsant serum levels: relationship to impairments of cognitive functioning. *J.Neurol.Neurosurg.Psych.*, **46**, 227–233.

TRIMBLE, M.R. and REYNOLDS, E.H. (1976) Anticonvulsant drugs and mental symptoms. *Psychol.Med.*, **6**, 169–174.

TRIMBLE, M.R. and THOMPSON, P.J. (1983) Anticonvulsant drugs, cognitive function, and behavior. *Epilepsia*, **24** (Suppl.1), S55–S63.

TURNER, W.A. (1907) *Epilepsy: a Study of the Idiopathic Disease*. Macmillan, London.

WECHSLER, D. (1944) *The Measurement of Adult Intelligence*, 3rd edition. Williams and Wilkins, Baltimore.

WECHSLER, D. (1945) A standardized memory scale for clinical use. *J.Psychol.*, **19**, 87–95.

WHITMORE, K. and HOLDSWORTH, L. (1971) Some observations from a study of children with epilepsy who were attending ordinary schools. *Spastic Society Study Group on Medical Aspects of Children with School Difficulties, Durham*.

YACORZYNSKI, G.K. and ARIEFF, A.J. (1942) Absence of deterioration in patients with non-organic epilepsy with especial reference to bromide therapy. *J.Nerv.Ment.Dis.*, **95**, 687–697.

3

Methods and problems in the assessment of behaviour disorders in epileptic patients

P.J. THOMPSON
The Chalfont Centre for Epilepsy, Chalfont St Peter, Buckinghamshire

INTRODUCTION

Behaviour disorder is a term used frequently but, unfortunately, variably. Some authors employ the term in a general way to encompass the main categories of psychiatric disturbance including psychosis, aggression, sexual dysfunction, affective disorder, personality and behaviour change, and general psychopathology (e.g. Hermann and Whitman, 1986). Others however use the term more narrowly as a distinct area of psychopathology and a subcategory of non-psychotic disorders, and within that category as separate from personality disorder, personality change and sexual dysfunction. Fenton (1981), who adopts the latter system, outlines the clinical features of a behaviour disorder as follows:

> irritability, moodiness and sometimes frank mood changes, social withdrawal, quarrelsomeness, and paranoid attitudes, temper tantrums and occasionally explosive aggressiveness, impulsiveness, restlessness, poor attention span, distractability and lack of application, disturbed inter-personal relationships and sometimes delinquent behaviour.

To avoid problems of definition a slightly different approach will be taken in this presentation. For behaviour to constitute a disorder it must deviate from some standard acceptable to the patient or individuals coming into contact with the patient. There may be an excess of an unwanted behaviour such as extreme explosions of temper. The behaviour itself may be normal but occurring in restricted or inappropriate contexts, e.g. removing clothes in public. Finally, a behaviour may be absent or poorly represented, for instance poor social skills and low self-esteem. According to this approach, behaviour characteristics

27

attributed by some to patients with epilepsy such as hypergraphia and religiosity (Fedio, 1986) would not be conceived of as behaviour disorders unless they were sufficiently severe to have a disruptive influence on an individual's life. Indeed some of these characteristics may actually have beneficial consequences depending on an individual's lifestyle and occupation.

In any discussion of methods and problems of assessment of behaviour disorders it becomes important to state the assessment goals. To date, the majority of studies of adults with epilepsy have attempted to classify and measure rates of behaviour problems in different groups. Comparisons have been made between patients with epilepsy and other disorders or between different types of seizure disorders. Studies of this nature have also explored the underlying factors contributing to behaviour disturbance (Hermann and Whitman, 1984, 1986). However, these studies will not be the subject of this chapter. It is other aims of assessment which have been relatively neglected in respect of epilepsy that will be considered, namely assessment for intervention and linked to this, assessment of the effectiveness of intervention.

In this evaluation of assessment methods, I shall draw upon my own experience with patients at the Chalfont Centre for Epilepsy. Many have intractable epilepsy, often with multiple seizure types and evidence of brain damage, and therefore constitute a high-risk group for behaviour disturbance (Hermann and Whitman 1984; Rodin, 1987). Over 300 patients have long-term placements. A survey of this group ($n=321$) in 1985 suggested considerable behaviour problems did exist. Problem behaviours were not objectively defined but included 'aggression, social withdrawal and antisocial habits'. Forty-six per cent were assessed to have problem behaviour and in 38% the behaviour was assessed by staff to constitute a management problem, defined as considerable care or supervision required constantly or occasionally. In addition patients pass through the Assessment Unit at the Chalfont Centre for Epilepsy. This Unit provides a full medical assessment of patients' epilepsy as well as examining employment potential and living skills. Most of these patients have uncontrollable or complicated epilepsy but they only remain at the Centre for four months and then are discharged. The case notes of 40 patients admitted during 1987 were scrutinized for evidence of any behaviour difficulties. Table 1 lists descriptions applied to 17 patients in this group. In the first few weeks of a patient's admission, staff rate behaviour on a scale which has been developed for use at the Chalfont Centre. Staff observations are used to evaluate a range of abilities and behaviours. Aspects measured include social behaviour, motivation, concentration, depression, anxiety, tiredness, irritability and insight. The scale itself is open to several methological criticisms outlined in the next section. However, staff ratings of a sample of patients admitted in 1987 suggest the most significant difficulties lie in the area of social behaviour and motivation, and the least problems are encountered in the area of tiredness and irritability.

Table 1.   Examples of behavoural problems attributed to assessment unit patients

---

Immature personality
Irresponsible behaviour
Temper tantrums
Aggressive, tormenting, rebellious
Physically aggressive
Violent outbursts
Verbal aggression
Suicidal attempts
Attention-seeking
Mood swings
Apathy

METHODS OF ASSESSMENT

Interview

This represents the most frequently used form of assessment of behaviour disorders. Interviews vary in the degree of structure imposed, but the unstructured interview is probably the most commonly employed form of assessment in the United Kingdom. A major aim of the interview is to obtain a clear account of the problem behaviour, in particular, what it is, when it happens and how frequently it happens. The interview may be with the person presenting with the behaviour disorder but more often with the types of problem discussed above, it is the family or staff for whom the behaviour is a problem and from whom information must be elicited. An attempt should be made to isolate the different events and situations associated with the behaviour; what occurs before and after difficult episodes including how individuals in the environment respond. Knowledge of the places in which the problems arise is useful. For instance, do they occur in the home setting and not in the work setting, or vice versa? In addition it is valuable to gain developmental information about the onset of problem behaviour and in particular what is going on in the life of the individual within the family, at work, and including any treatment alterations or changes in the control of seizures.

In epilepsy, the temporal relationship of the problem behaviours to seizures should always be explored. Occasionally what is described as a problem behaviour in the interview by a family may be an actual seizure, or be occurring in the postictal phase of the attack (Fenton, 1986). A patient's knowledge and attitude to his epilepsy may also underlie behaviour problems. Mittan and colleagues have provided evidence that stress can arise as a result of a patient's fears and misconceptions about the seizures. For instance, they report from their survey that 70% of individuals express a fear of dying in their next seizure and many individuals seemed almost housebound due to a fear of having a seizure (Mittan, 1986). Often the family's understanding of, and attitude to, epilepsy may need to be explored. It is not uncommon to find beliefs such as reprimands or too much stress will 'bring on a seizure'. Misunderstandings about the disorder may result in too many restrictions being placed upon the individual. Patients with epilepsy may be restricted from activities that their contemporaries take for granted. Some individuals are not left alone or allowed to move from an armchair if family members are not present. This can occur in very extreme forms, indeed one family recently encountered kept a constant vigil of their son while he was in hospital and refused to have him home for fear he would die in a seizure. Another father made no attempt to reprimand or restrain his adult son for aggressive acts because he believed this was all part of having epilepsy and to be expected. The problem behaviour may arise not through restrictions on the individual *per se* but in addition through restrictions that the family experience on their lifestyle which can make families socially isolated (Lechtenberg, 1984). Ignorance surrounding epilepsy may also extend to nursing and other care staff.

Total reliance on information obtained from an interview is generally unwise. It is sometimes difficult to establish the accuracy of such information and this decreases the reliability of this technique. Further, it is often difficult to get families or staff to give specific descriptions of problem behaviour that are devoid of inferential statements such as 'attention-seeking'.

Questionnaires

Questionnaires and inventories are generally viewed as being more objective and standardized than an interview. Many measures available are quick and inexpensive to administer in terms of staff time and material (Jensen and Haynes, 1986). The content of such questionnaires can vary considerably. The most structured and widely-used techniques in the field of epilepsy are personality inventories such as the Minnesota Multiphasic Personality Inventory (MMPI: Dodrill and Batzel, 1986). Such measures can be adopted to provide diagnostic labels and may be of limited value when assessment is undertaken to devise an intervention. Other measures are available which provide information about an individual's mood, for instance the Beck Depression Inventory (Beck et al., 1961); the Spielberger Scales of anxiety (Spielberger, 1975); and the Hospital Anxiety and Depression (HAD) Scale (Zigmond and Snaith, 1983). These scales may provide important information that influences subsequent intervention. The Bear-Fedio questionnaire, reported as being developed especially to detect behaviour changes in epilepsy, remains controversial (Rodin and Schmaltz, 1984).

Over the last ten to fifteen years many more problem-orientated questionnaires have been developed to assess specific behaviour such as social skills or fears. Many are constructed with the aim of assessment for intervention (e.g.

Cohen-Conger and Conger 1986; Jensen and Haynes, 1986). Such techniques may be idiosyncratic to a particular assessment centre or assessor and even within assessment centres they may be specific to a particular patient. The assessment ratings of behaviours made by nursing staff at the Chalfont Centre fall into this category and are therefore open to all the criticisms made against such unstandardized measures (see below).

The usefulness of assessment techniques can be measured with respect to their dependability and generalizability. These characteristics have been most extensively investigated with respect to questionnaires and a voluminous literature exists on ways of assessing the reliability and validity of such measures (Anastasi, 1982; Sechrest, 1984; Jensen and Haynes, 1986). Measures of reliability include the stability of a measuring instrument over time (test-retest reliability) and the stability between raters (inter-rater reliability). Measures that are influenced by practice effects and reactivity will have a low test-retest reliability, but also, when genuine changes in behaviour have occurred between two test administrations, this will also result in a low reliability coefficient.

The validity of a test can be measured in various ways. A test is said to have face validity if it looks as if it is measuring what it claims to measure. Another important form of validity is concurrent validity where scores on a newly developed test are correlated with some known standard for the particular construct being assessed. Concurrent validity estimates are beset by problems concerning criteria against which to assess a new test. For example, if one assesses the validity of a questionnaire by using another established questionnaire then there is a possibility that a high correlation may simply be reflecting the similarity in testing method and not content of the measure. Furthermore, if a measure correlates highly with another technique and it cannot be demonstrated that any additional information stems from employing the new measure then it will have low incremental validity. The majority of questionnaires which can be used for assessment to plan an intervention have limited data available on their reliability and validity. This is certainly the case for many of the assessment measures employed at the Chalfont Centre, however I would argue that this does not necessarily detract from their usefulness, particularly when they are being used to plan interventions and assess the value of any treatments undertaken.

A lack of normative information is a further criticism that can be levelled against many questionnaires. This is particularly a problem in the assessment of behaviour disorders. Without normative data it may be difficult to establish what are reasonable goals to aim for. We may set our goals too high, and above behaviour found in the individual's peer group. Normative data may also be useful in establishing the clinical significance of any behaviour change. The importance of normative data has been highlighted recently in the assessment of social skills. Here many questionnaires have been developed to rate behaviour and many have been shown to have high reliability and validity. Unfortunately much work has involved university students – a very select group – and therefore the relevance of norms developed in this way is unclear (Cohen-Conger and Conger, 1986). Social desirability is an additional problem that can arise with questionnaires. Respondents may wish to present themselves in a favourable light and this may result in an under-reporting of negative behaviour and over-reporting of positive behaviour. Some questionnaires incorporate into their scales techniques to reduce this effect, for example the use of lie scales. Dodrill et al. (1980) employed such a technique in the Washington Psychosocial Inventory (WPSI). A high score on the lie scale invalidates the responses made to the other questions. Unfortunately this can result in a significant loss of data. In an unpublished study of psychosocial functioning in patients from the Assessment Unit at Chalfont, a quarter of the WPSI questionnaires had to be excluded from the analysis due to elevated lie scores.

Finally, two further disadvantages of many existing questionnaires encountered with the patient group referred to in this chapter deserve consideration. Some questionnaires take considerable time to administer and score and this greatly reduces their practical value. Patients with limited ability and literacy skills may not adequately understand all of the questions, and naturally this reduces the value of several measures currently available.

Self-monitoring

A variety of procedures including diaries, mechanical counters, daily charts and portable monitoring devices, exists to obtain self-observation data. A decision to use a particular procedure is determined by such factors as ease with which the targeted symptom can be detected by the patient, symptom frequency, the intellectual ability of the patient, and the degree of interference posed by the particular procedure given a patient's daily routine. These methods can be particularly useful in gaining baseline information about the frequency of certain behaviours which cannot be observed readily, or monitored easily by other individuals. (Bornstein et al., 1986). I have found these methods to be useful and they can be adapted for individuals of quite limited ability.

One mentally handicapped patient was referred because she was experiencing significant distress because of disturbing thoughts at night which kept her awake. The thought involved was that 'her head was going to fall off'. Obviously such thoughts could not be observed by others. Self-monitoring involved placing a symbol in a modified diary to indicate if the thoughts had been experienced the night before. This technique yielded useful baseline information which was used to assess the efficacy of a thought-stopping intervention programme (Rimm and Masters, 1979). Another patient of limited ability was referred to me for 'extreme apathy'. One particular aspect of this problem which could be easily monitored was time of getting up. The individual was encouraged to record this on a daily basis with staff signing his record as an accuracy check.

Issues of reliability and validity again arise with these measuring techniques. Self-monitoring is dependent on the accuracy of the patient. Furthermore if the demands of self-observation are high, requiring the completion of diaries every evening or several times a day, then compliance may also be a problem reducing the usefulness of this technique. In studies which have assessed the agreement between observer and subjective monitoring there have been widely discrepant accuracy results, ranging from near-perfect agreement in some studies to total lack of agreement in others. Bornstein et al. (1986) comment: 'self-monitoring when used as an assessment technique clearly demands accurate and unbiased self-reporting. Unfortunately such accuracy is more the exception than the rule.' Seizure documentation by patients invariably relies on self-monitoring and often is the measure which is employed to judge the efficacy of treatment. The reliability of this form of self-monitoring has been the subject of little investigation.

A further problem of self-monitoring frequently cited is the reactivity of this technique. The very operation of self-monitoring can result in changes in the target behaviour. For this reason it can be difficult in some instances to get accurate baselines. While such reactive effects compromise the assessment functions of this measure they can be of substantial therapeutic value in the remediation of problem behaviour. For the patient mentioned above with problems of motivation, the act of self-monitoring has proved a useful adjunct to treatment. Recording the times he has risen seems to have contributed to an improvement in his behaviour. On the two occasions when this self-monitoring was discontinued his behaviour deteriorated and improvement occurred with the reintroduction of the self-monitoring device. He has now been using this self-monitoring technique for over three years!

Direct observation

Direct observation procedures can be classified into simulated observation and observation in natural settings. The former are specifically constructed to evoke a sample of behaviour. The most popular method is role play. In this situation the participants act through a particular situation. It may be a useful technique for low frequency events which can be prompted easily. Furthermore it is possible to record an individual's behaviour, either by audiotape or preferably by videotape which can allow more detailed assessment. Major problems however do exist with such techniques, for instance while a role play situation can seem to be reflecting actual situations in the natural world this cannot be presumed. Individuals may be very aware of the artificiality of the situation and may behave very differently when role playing. These techniques are frequently used with patients at the Chalfont Centre for Epilepsy particularly as part of social skills programmes. A concern expressed by staff is this discrepancy between performance in the simulated situation and that encountered in more natural surroundings.

Direct observation in natural settings can be a valuable source of information. A variety of recording procedures exists, the selection of which often depends on the nature of the presenting problem behaviour. These will not be discussed in detail here but include continuous recording, frequency recording, durational recording, time sampling and interval recording. (For review see Ciminero et al., 1986). Descriptions of these procedures suggest accuracy is improved by having clear objective descriptions of behaviour, for instance in recording the frequency of social interactions between patients in a group then the preferred description would be of the format 'an audible verbalization comprised of words with an eye directed at another individual'. These objective descriptions are believed to reduce inferences necessary on the part of the observer. In accounts given of direct observation it is suggested that accuracy will be improved by having trained observers who do not participate in any way in the observed scene. Strict guidelines are often given regarding the characteristics of a reliable observer, the training required and how frequently to make accuracy checks on the recordings they make. Following such guidelines generally necessitates significant resources including additional highly trained personnel which are generally not available in most clinic settings.

For observational data on behaviour disorders it is generally necessary to rely on recordings by family members or by care staff. It is necessary to reduce the demands of the technique by ensuring that the sampling procedures are easy to follow and, more importantly, they do not significantly interfere with the other demands made upon the staff time or family life. In this way reliability and validity of the technique may be compromised. However, observational data of this form can be useful in providing information such as the relationship of behaviours to seizures.

Neuropsychological assessment

Patients with epilepsy most likely to present with behaviour difficulties generally have difficult-to-control seizures and evidence of underlying brain damage (Rodin, 1987). These patients are also at risk for deficits of cognitive functioning and for intellectual deterioration (Trimble and Thompson, 1986; Thompson et al., 1987). Evidence exists suggesting that neuropsychological impairment is not an uncommon accompaniment of emotional and psychiatric problems and that in some instances it may underlie the disturbance of the patient (Hermann and Whitman, 1986). Neuropsychological assessments undertaken on patients at the Chalfont Centre for Epilepsy do reveal a high level of cognitive disturbance. A recent investigation of 50 longstay residents

Table 2.   Percentage of patients from the residential population with cognitive deficits (N = 50)

Test areas	Degree of impairments		
	None	Moderate	Severe
Visual perception	62	28	10
Memory	8	54	38
Language	46	48	6
Frontal lobe functioning	38	14	48

who were being given training to improve independent living skills revealed major neuropsychological deficits (Table 2). Furthermore, it is common to find patients from the Assessment Unit mislabelled as mentally handicapped and who are presenting problems that are in part a response to their undemanding environment. Conversely, individuals may have too high expectations placed upon them and these can underlie behaviour problems. Neuropsychological information, when combined with data of a more observational nature, can be very informative regarding reasons for difficult behaviour.

Additional methods

Medical and social records often provide valuable information in the assessment of behaviour problems. Besides providing a quick reference for many demographic facts, they may point to important antecedent events and reinforcers of difficult behaviours. Particular note should be taken of possible medication changes which may coincide with the onset of difficult behaviour or deterioration in seizure control or other significant changes in lifestyle or life events that may have occurred.

A valuable instrument in the evaluation of behaviour problems particularly when these have been unexplained by other assessments is the EEG (Fenwick, Chapter 5). The conventional EEG recording is somewhat limited because recordings are undertaken in artificial conditions, remote from the environment in which the problem behaviours occur. More valuable information may be obtained via ambulatory monitoring using a miniature tape recorder. This technique permits long-term recording for periods of a day or longer in natural environments. Video telemetry is another technique that may be useful, although the nature of the recording results in a certain degree of artificiality. These techniques are considered at greater length in Chapters 4 and 5.

When behaviour disturbance is acute in onset or inconsistent with past behaviour, the measurement of antiepileptic drug serum levels may be valuable. Patients may be more likely to present with problems when drug levels are high, particularly in the toxic range (Reynolds, 1986).

AGGRESSIVE BEHAVIOUR

The association between aggressive behaviour and epilepsy has a long history. Fortunately more recent studies with improved methodology demonstrate that aggressive behaviour is not as widespread as previously assumed. Fenwick (1986) writes; 'The age-old stigma attached to the majority of epileptics as being aggressive impulsive people finds little support in scientific study.' Referral from the residential sample at the Chalfont Centre because of aggressive behaviour is an infrequent occurrence, but when such behaviours arise they can present significant management problems and they do necessitate some form of intervention. In this final section I hope to demonstrate via three case-studies how careful assessment using some of the methods discussed above can highlight certain causes and factors contributing to aggressive presentations in patients with epilepsy.

Case study 1

Carol is 34 years old and had been a resident at the Chalfont Centre for twelve years at the time of referral. The age of onset of her seizures is not clear but is presumed to have occurred in childhood. On admission to Chalfont she was described as emotionally disturbed and it was thought that many of her seizures were psychological in origin. Her behaviour had failed to respond to treatment with antidepressants and major tranquillizers. Assessments of her attacks in 1975 suggested that a number were indeed epileptic and a right frontal focus was recorded on her EEG. Antiepileptic medication was adjusted and there was significant improvement in her behaviour. For several years she was not reported as presenting any management problems. She was referred in 1985 because of temper outbursts which on occasion involved injury to other patients. Her assessment involved self-monitoring of her outbursts of temper, observations by staff, scrutinization of case records, an EEG and blood level monitoring. There was no association between her difficult behaviour and seizures, indeed she was experiencing good seizure control at the time. There had been no recent medication changes and all serum levels were similar within the therapeutic range and at levels which she had previously tolerated. Self-monitoring revealed that outbursts of aggression only occurred in her 'home environment' and never when she was working. At that time she undertook secretarial duties in the Appeals Department of the Centre. Psychological assessment revealed an individual of average ability with no significant cognitive difficulties. Rating scales of mood revealed her to be moderately depressed and she was preoccupied with a fear of mental deterioration. A major factor underlying her difficult behaviour seemed to be her living conditions. In fact, she was significantly more able than the majority of residents in her home environment. Staff frequently expected her help to assist the other less able residents and were very disapproving when she was not eager to do so. She was aware that a number of her living companions were deteriorating mentally and physically. The assessment suggested that she was wrongly placed and also that she had cognitive resources to exert some influence on her difficult behaviour. A subsequent move to a higher-level environment and short-term psychotherapeutic intervention focusing on strategies to control temper have resulted in no further difficult behaviour.

Case study 2

Joyce is a 53-year-old woman who had been a resident at the Chalfont Centre for three years. She was assessed to have complex partial seizures with left a frontotemporal focus. She was referred because of verbal aggression and irritability which staff felt was having a detrimental influence on her relationship with them and other residents. They also expressed the belief that although she was considered to be a fairly difficult individual, at times her behaviour was particularly intolerable. A psychological assessment revealed no specific cognitive deficts, no depression or undue anxiety, furthermore she lacked insight into her difficult behaviour. There had been no significant changes in her medication dose or in her seizure control to coincide with the reported difficult behaviour. Staff observations of her behaviour have been undertaken at intervals over more than a year. This has involved a 7-point rating of her level of irritability. The patient also completed rating scales of mood and tests of concentration over this period. Her anticonvulsant serum levels and seizure frequency were monitored. Her serum levels were always recorded above the therapeutic range, and on the occasions when the serum level was particularly high her behaviour was rated by staff to be most problematic. Unfortunately, attempts to reduce her medication on two occasions have resulted in an exacerbation of seizures during which she has sustained significant injuries. Her behaviour at times continues to be a problem but it may be possible, with exploration of alternative medication, that some improvements will occur.

Case study 3

Deborah is a 22-year-old patient who was admitted to the Assessment Unit at the Chalfont Centre for Epilepsy. She has experienced complex partial seizures from early infancy with no significant periods of remission. EEGs have revealed a left mid-temporal focus. Her family background was very unsettled. She was born illegitimate with a Greek Cypriot father. Her mother subsequently married another individual and the family moved to the West Indies. At the age of four years she was sent to live with her grandmother because it was felt her epilepsy could be better treated in England. She has a history of social and psychological deprivation. Behaviour problems have been frequently documented including temper tantrums. Observations by staff revealed that aggression was not a feature of her behaviour during her stay at the Assessment Unit. However, significant periods of postictal confusion upwards of 20 minutes were recorded, and if intervention by staff was attempted during this time then she would hit out and become verbally abusive. Neuropsychological assessment revealed significant receptive and expressive language deficits. These factors were felt to have contributed to her recorded past difficult behaviour although her psychologically and social unstable background may have resulted in past assessments focusing on reasons such as rejection by the family and inconsistent handling as underlying her difficult behaviours.

CONCLUSIONS

Method and problems in the assessment of behaviour disorders in epilepsy have been discussed with particular reference to patients with intractable epilepsy, a high-risk group for behaviour disturbance. The aim has been to review methods of assessment which may prove valuable for devising intervention plans. Methods fulfilling this role have been neglected in the past relative to measures aimed at classifying and estimating the incidence of behaviour disorders. Nevertheless, the approaches discussed, although often lacking appropriate standardization, may be useful. The three cases of aggressive behaviour outlined demonstrate the multifactorial nature of behaviour problems and, more importantly, that assessment can result in interventions which reduce or eliminate such management difficulties. Unfortunately, there still exists a lack of understanding about epilepsy that leads some professionals and families to accept difficult behaviour as part of the epileptic condition. More investigations into the assessment and non-pharmacological treatment of difficult behaviour in patients with epilepsy seems worthwhile and to be of direct relevance to those individuals who care for patients with problematic epilepsy.

REFERENCES

ANASTASI, A. (1982) *Psychological Testing*, 5th edition. Macmillan, New York.
BECK, A.T., WARD, C.H., MENDELSON, M., MOCK, J. and ERBAUGH, J. (1961) An inventory for measuring depression. *Arch.Gen.Psychiat.*, **4**, 561–571.
BORNSTEIN, P.B., HAMILTON, S.B. and BORNSTEIN, M.T. (1986) Self-monitoring procedures. In *Handbook of Behavioural Assessment* 2nd edition (eds. A.R. CIMINERO, K.S. CALHOUN and H.E. ADAMS), pp. 176–222. John Wiley & Sons, New York.
CIMINERO, A.R., CALHOUN, K.S. and ADAMS, H.E. (1986) *Handbook of Behavioural Assessment*, 2nd edition. John Wiley & Sons, New York.
COHEN-COHEN, J. and CONGER, A.J. (1986) Assessment of social skills. In *Handbook of Behavioural Assessment*, 2nd edition, pp. 526–560 (eds A.R. CIMINERO, K.S. CALHOUN and H.G. ADAMS). John Wiley & Sons, New York.

DODRILL, C.B. and BATZEL, L.W. (1986) Interictal behavioural features of patients with epilepsy. *Epilepsia*, **27** (Suppl.2), 564–576.

DODRILL, C.B., BATZEL, L.W., QUEISSER, H.R. and TEMKIN, N.R. (1980) An objective method for assessment of psychological and social problems among epileptics. *Epilepsia*, **21**, 123–135.

FEDIO, P. (1986) Behavioural characteristics of temporal lobe epilepsy. *Psychiatr. Am. North Am.*, **9**, 283–292.

FENTON, G.W. (1981) Psychiatric disorders of epilepsy: classification and phenomenology. In *Epilepsy and Psychiatry* (eds E.H. REYNOLDS and M.R. TRIMBLE), pp. 12–26. Churchill-Livingstone, New York.

FENTON, G.W. (1986) The EEG epilepsy and psychiatry. In *What is Epilepsy? The Clinical Scientific Basis of Epilepsy* (eds M.R. TRIMBLE and E.H. REYNOLDS), pp. 139–160. Churchill-Livingstone, Edinburgh.

FENWICK, P. (1986) Aggression and epilepsy. In *Aspects of Epilepsy and Psychiatry* (eds M.R. TRIMBLE and T.G. BOLWIG), pp. 31–57. John Wiley & Sons, Chichester.

HERMANN, B.P. and WHITMAN, S. (1984) Behavioural and personality correlates of epilepsy: a review, methodological critique and conceptual model. *Psych.Bull.*, **95**, 451–497.

HERMANN, B.P. and WHITMAN, S. (1986) Psychopathology in epilepsy: a multifactiological model. In *Psychopathology in Epilepsy Social Dimensions* (eds S. WHITMAN and B.P. HERMANN), pp. 5–37. Oxford University Press, New York.

JENSEN, B.J. and HAYNES, S.N. (1986) Self-report questionnaires and inventories. In *Handbook of Behavioural Assessment*, 2nd edition, pp. 150–175 (eds A.R. CIMINERO, K.S. CALHOUN and H.E. ADAMS). John Wiley & Sons, New York.

LECHTENBERG, R. (1984) *Epilepsy and the Family*. Harvard University Press, Cambridge, Massachusetts.

MITTAN, R.J. (1986) Fear of seizures. In *Psychopathology in Epilepsy: Social Dimensions* (eds S. WHITMAN and B.P. HERMANN), pp. 90–121. Oxford University Press, New York.

REYNOLDS, E.H. (1986) Antiepileptic drugs and personality. In *Aspects of Epilepsy and Psychiatry* (eds M.R. TRIMBLE and T.G. BOLWIG), pp. 89–99. John Wiley & Sons, Chichester.

RIMM, D.C. and MASTERS, J.C. (1979) *Behaviour Therapy: Techniques and Empirical Findings*. Academic Press, New York.

RODIN, E. (1987) Factors which influence prognosis in epilepsy. In *Epilepsy* (ed. A. HOPKINS), pp.339–371. Chapman & Hall, London.

RODIN, E. and SCHMALTZ, S. (1984) The Bear–Fedio Inventory and Temporal Lobe Epilepsy. *Neurology*, **34**, 591–596.

SECHREST, L. (1984) Reliability and validity. In *Research Methods in Clinical Psychology* (eds A.S. BELLACK and M. HERSEN), pp. 24–54. Pergamon Press, New York.

SPIELBERGER, C.D. (1975) The measurement of state and trait anxiety: conceptual and methodological issues. In *Emotions – Their Parameters and Measurement* (ed. L. LEVI), pp. 713–725. Raven Press, New York.

THOMPSON, P.J., SANDER, J.W.A.S. and OXLEY, J. (1987) Intellectual deterioration in severe epilepsy. In *Advances in Epileptology*, Vol.16 (eds P. WOLF, M. DAN, D. JANZAND, and F.G. DREIFUSS), pp. 611–614. Raven Press, New York.

TRIMBLE, M.R. and THOMPSON, P.J. (1986) Neuropsychology of epilepsy and its treatment. In *Neuropsychological Assessment of Neuropsychiatric Disorders* (eds I. GRANT and K.M. ADAMS), pp. 321–346. Oxford University Press, New York.

ZIGMOND, A.S. and SNAITH, R.P. (1983) The hospital anxiety and depression scale. *Acta Psychiat. Scand.*, **67**, 361–370.

Discussion

Section I

Professor J.A. Corbett: Dr Thompson discussed categories of cognitive or behavioural impairment, some of which were described by functions, for example, perceptual, but one was 'frontal'. Do you think that it is helpful to describe problems in terms of site of origin, rather than functionally? 'Frontal' almost seems at times to be used as a pejorative term like 'psychopath' or 'hysteria'.

Dr P.J. Thompson: The term frontal is used because it conveys what other people may call executive functions, to do with organizing and planning. It's just a convenient summary term. I am not necessarily using it in an anatomical localizing sense. I would rather refer to the disorders of the function that give rise to behavioural problems. I would rather use the term 'memory' than for example 'temporal lobe problems'.

Dr M.R. Trimble: This is a very important issue, because if you confuse two classifications, one of which is clinical and the other anatomical, you run into semantic and conceptual problems. I get meaningless referrals saying 'This patient has had an aggressive outburst. Is this temporal lobe epilepsy or is it a behavioural disorder?' This is tautology. The term 'frontal', I think, ought to be applied to an anatomical/pathological definition.

Dr S.H. Green (Birmingham): Can you comment on assessment of children, especially in an outpatient setting?

Ms J. Ossetin: We use the Conner's and Rutter's Behavioural Questionnaires, which have two parallel forms, for parents and for teachers. Parents complete the forms at the same time as their child is being assessed. The teacher's questionnaires are sent off together with an accompanying letter to the head of the school and to the child's teacher. In the letters we invite the school to contact us for further explanation and information, or for advice if the child has any problems. We spend time going to the school and discussing problems with the teachers who like to be involved. I have also been to the homes of some of the children and talked with the parents. There is often a degree of over-protection but people are sometimes very cooperative and take advice given.

Dr F.M.C. Besag: The over-protection syndrome is something very primitive in the parents, which is not very amenable to rational argument. It is very important for carers to recognize this phenomenon.

We have found that verbal–performance discrepancies in both directions can be associated with behavioural disorders in our children. The person who has either a comprehension difficulty or an expressive difficulty with better performance than verbal abilities, not surprisingly, may become very frustrated and can show aggressive outbursts. They are not able to express their frustrations verbally. The other group, who have better verbal abilities than performance abilities, we, as professionals punish. They sit in our clinics and we think, well you're presenting yourself very well, why don't you get on with your life? They simply can't because they are presenting themselves much better than they can perform; we are judging them on what they say and not on what they are actually able to do. I think verbal–performance discrepancies in both directions are very important for us to take note of when we are assessing our patients.

Dr C. Verity (Cambridge): Ms Ossetin, you have nicely reviewed the difficulties of studying cognitive function in groups of patients. Parents and teachers are often worried about individual children and they want to know whether we think that drugs are responsible for cognitive deficits. Do you think that any of the tests which are available are useful in this respect?

Ms J. Ossetin: Many of these tests are useful, but we do not know how much change in performance has to occur for it to be significant. We are in need of normative data. Motor-pursuits tasks, like space invader games, and tests of attentional span are sensitive to drug effects. Further, the more complicated the tasks the greater the drug related impairment. However, if you make tasks complicated, you do not really know which element of that task is impaired.

Dr. P.B.C. Fenwick: Dr Reynolds, do you feel that psychiatrists or neurologists are the people to treat epileptic patients?

Dr E.H. Reynolds: The clinicians who treat epilepsy should be those who are interested in treating epilepsy, whether paedatricians or neurologists or psychiatrists. I do not think that you and I should spend too much time passing patients backwards and forwards between each other. You are perfectly competent to deal with most of the neurological aspects and I feel that I have learnt enough to deal with many of the psychological aspects. Epilepsy does not belong exclusively to psychiatry or neurology but to physicians who take a special interest in it. Of course, problems do arise which require special expertise and one may want to call in the paediatric neurologist or the psychiatrist for some cases. In general, however, I think one should be an 'all-rounder'. This is a principle that applies to medicine as a whole.

I pointed out that historically there has been much division of opinion between neurologists and psychiatrists for a number of reasons, including the separation of neurology from psychiatry, and the fact that neurologists and psychiatrists have different perspectives because they see different patients. That is not to say that I wish to see this process continue. Far from it. It is possible now, I think, for neurologists and psychiatrists to see things in similar ways.

Section II

4

Seizures, EEG discharges and cognition

COLIN D. BINNIE
The Maudsley Hospital, London

TRANSITORY COGNITIVE IMPAIRMENT

Although the occurrence of abnormal neuronal discharges is fundamental to current concepts of epilepsy, the clinical significance or otherwise of interictal epileptiform EEG discharges has long been a subject of controversy. The occurrence of generalized spike-wave activity during absence seizures was one of the first discoveries of clinical electroencephalography, yet it was soon realized that such discharges were not necessarily accompanied by any clinical manifestations (Gibbs et al., 1936). Such discharges came to be described as 'subclinical' or 'larval'. However, this concept too had shortly to be modified when Schwab (1939) showed that when patients performed a simple reaction time task during EEG monitoring, subclinical spike-wave discharges might be accompanied by slowed reactions or a complete failure to respond. Since that time some 40 further studies have confirmed the occurrence of transitory cognitive impairment (TCI) during generalized subclinical EEG discharges, both in patients who appeared to be seizure-free and even in people not thought to have epilepsy (Ishihara and Yoshii, 1967). This extensive literature has been reviewed elsewhere (Binnie, 1980; Aarts et al., 1984). Overall most investigators have found TCI in roughly half the patients studied, however, the demonstration of TCI depends both on the psychological test employed and the nature of the EEG discharges. Intellectually demanding tasks, particularly ones demanding high rates of information handling, are most likely to demonstrate TCI. By contrast, simple repetitive motor or mental tasks, such as tapping, counting, recitation, or operation of a pursuit rotor, and indeed simple reaction time as studied by Schwab, are relatively insensitive to the effects of subclinical discharges.

The EEG phenomena themselves may be crucial determinants: TCI is most often demonstrable during prolonged, generalized, symmetrical, regular, spike-wave discharges at about three per second. The less the EEG phenomena correspond to this stereotype, the less likely is TCI to be found. Until recently (Aarts et al., 1984), there were no documented reports of TCI during focal discharges. It is sometimes possible to demonstrate a progressive impairment of cognition developing over the first one or two seconds of a prolonged discharge with recovery shortly before the abnormal EEG activity ceases, a so-called 'trough of consciousness' (Browne et al., 1974). It was widely reported that discharges of less than 3 seconds' duration were unlikely to produce a demonstrable TCI.

DETECTING TCI

Investigation of TCI presents some practical difficulties. Few patients exhibit prolonged subclinical EEG discharges in the alert, eyes open state more often than, say, once per minute, unless also suffering frequent overt seizures. During attention to a difficult task, epileptiform activity often becomes less frequent, so that it may be difficult to capture during a period of testing acceptable to the patient a sufficient number of discharges to form any reliable conclusion about the occurrence of TCI. The advent of microcomputer graphics has provided a solution however, as it is now possible to disguise continuous psychological tasks as agreeable television games, which patients are prepared to play for periods sufficient to allow capture of large numbers of discharges. Aarts et al. (1984) report the use of two such games incorporating a short-term memory task, the one requiring recall of spatial information, the other using verbal material. These computer-controlled tasks were adaptive, the difficulty being automatically adjusted to the highest level of performance which the patient could achieve.

Apparently this method of testing was of greater sensitivity than those previously used; for instance, it demonstrated TCI during focal discharges, which had not previously been achieved. Moreover, the authors were at pains to monitor behaviour throughout the investigation by CCTV, and they excluded all subjects demonstrating overt clinical seizures during the test. The application of this criterion was found to eliminate all patients with generalized regular 3 per second spike-wave discharges of 3 seconds' duration or longer. Yet despite exclusion of just those subjects in whom others had most readily demonstrated TCI, they were able to demonstrate cognitive impairment in 50% of their patients (Table 1).

A further original finding was an interaction between the nature of the task and lateralization of discharges. In patients with focal or markedly asymmetrical discharges, it was found that these were more likely to produce impairment of the spatial task if lateralized to the right and of the verbal task if left-sided. This effect, which was highly significant, was confirmed in a larger

Table 1. Effect of discharges on performance

Subjects with demonstrable TCI

Discharge type	Spatial task	Verbal task	Either or both tasks
Generalized	17/39 (44%)	9/32 (28%)	21/42 (50%)
Max./focal right	12/21 (57%)	2†/19 (11%)	12/21 (57%)
Max./focal left	4/27 (15%)	9/26 (35%)	13/29 (45%)
All types*	32/86 (37%)	19/73 (26%)	45/91 (49%)

* One patient had both right- and left-sided discharges.
† Includes 1 left-handed patient.
Reprinted with permission from Binnie et al. (1987).

series by Binnie et al. (1987) (Table 1), and has been independently verified by Rugland et al. (1987).

TCI AND NEUROPSYCHOLOGICAL TESTING

This last finding has interesting theoretical implications. It had hitherto been assumed that TCI involved a global impairment of vigilance or attention or a reduction in the brain's overall rate of transmission of information (Hutt et al., 1977). The apparent specificity of the site (or at least the side) of discharge to the nature of the cognitive impairment shows this interpretation to be inadequate. Moreover, it suggests that subclinical EEG discharges may contribute to selective deficits found when neuropsychological test batteries are applied to persons with epilepsy. Although it is well established (Dodrill and Wilkus, 1976) that abnormal psychological test profiles are more likely to be found in persons with frequent subclinical EEG discharges, the causality of this relationship is uncertain. EEG abnormality and cognitive deficits could both reflect the underlying pathology, or the type and severity of the epilepsy. However, continuous EEG recording during psychological testing allows the instantaneous effects of discharges on individual test items to be studied.

A recent study by Siebelink et al. (1988) addresses this issue. The shortened version of the revised Amsterdam Children's Intelligence Test was administered to a group of 21 schoolchildren with epilepsy, under continuous EEG and video monitoring. As a group, they exhibited an abnormal test profile with selective impairment on a subtest involving short-term verbal memory. However, this anomalous profile was shown only by those children who exhibited subclinical discharges during the test in question. Item-by-item analysis of the relationship between the occurrence of discharges and of errors showed a significant positive association on four of the six sub-tests and it appeared that the anomalous test profile could be explained by the particular sensitivity of the short-term verbal memory test to the effects of subclinical discharges.

This result has interesting implications for the interpretation of neuro-psychological findings in epilepsy. For instance, in pre-operative assessment neuropsychological evidence of damage in a particular region of the brain is regarded as offering independent corroboration of EEG localization. If the neuropsychological deficits are in fact attributable to the localized EEG disturbance then the two are clearly not independent.

PRACTICAL IMPLICATIONS OF TCI

Few investigators who have studied TCI appear to have addressed its possible practical consequences for day-to-day cognitive functioning. Yet the therapeutic implications of subclinical EEG discharges are a matter of concern and controversy for many clinicians. If, for instance, a child who is performing badly at school exhibits episodic cerebral dysfunction as evidenced by the EEG, it may seem reasonable to some that a trial of anticonvulsants should be carried out in the hope that this will improve cognitive functioning. Others will take the contrary view that an EEG disturbance is not a clinical manifestation and that antiepileptic drugs should be used only to suppress overt seizures. In fact the dispute centres on the definition of an epileptic seizure: it may be argued that an episodic impairment of cognition is a clinical manifestation and if it accompanies a cerebral dysrhythmia it meets current definitions of an epileptic seizure.

Ignoring the semantic debate, it may be more useful to consider whether subclinical discharges adversely affect the performance of day-to-day tasks. Kasteleijn et al. (1988) administered tests of educational skills to a group of 20 children under continuous EEG and video monitoring. Both during and immediately following subclinical discharges there was a statistically significant increase in the rate of errors whilst reading. It is difficult to avoid the conclusion that this observation is relevant to the classroom performance of children with such discharges.

More dramatically perhaps, Kasteleijn et al. (1987) performed telemetric EEG monitoring in a group of six patients with sub-clinical discharges whilst driving a motor vehicle. All were experienced motorists holding a current licence (although two still had active epilepsy). Driving performance was closely monitored by transducers attached to the test vehicle. Three of the six patients showed a statistically significant increase in the standard deviation of lateral road position in association with discharges; that is when discharges occurred they veered from side to side or failed to follow the curves of the road. It was not the purpose of this study to argue that persons with subclinical discharges are unfit to drive, but rather to highlight the relevance of TCI for the performance of everyday skills.

Individual patients are on record as having shown a worthwhile improvement of cognitive functioning and social adaptation when subclinical discharges were suppressed by antiepileptic drugs (Aarts et al., 1984). Whether an indication for treatment exists in only a small minority, or in many people with subclinical discharges, is unknown nor are any criteria established for identifying such patients. The need for further research in this area is obvious and urgent.

REFERENCES

AARTS, J.H.P., BINNIE, C.D., SMIT, A.M. and WILKINS, A.J. (1984) Selective cognitive impairment during focal and generalised epileptiform EEG activity. *Brain*, **107**, 293–308.

BINNIE, C.D. (1980). Detection of transitory cognitive impairment during epileptiform EEG discharges: problems in clinical practice. In *Epilepsy and Behaviour 1979* (Ed. B.M. KULIG, H. MEINARDI and G. STORES). Lisse: Swets and Zeitlinger, pp. 91–97.

BINNIE, C.D., KASTELEIJN-NOLST TRENITÉ, D.G.A., Smit, A.M. and Wilkins, A.J. (1987) Interactions of epileptiform EEG discharges and cognition. *Epilepsy Res.*, **1**, 239–245.

BROWNE, T.R., PENRY, J.K., PORTER, R.J. and DREIFUSS, F.E. (1974) Responsiveness before, during and after spike-wave paroxysms. *Neurology (Minneapolis)*, **24**, 659–665.

DODRILL, C.B. and WILKUS, R.J. (1976). Relationships between intelligence and electroencephalographic epileptiform activity in adult epileptics. *Neurology (Minneapolis)*, **26**, 525–531.

GIBBS, F.A., LENNOX, W.G. and GIBBS, E.L. (1936) The electroencephalogram in diagnosis and in localisation of epileptic seizures. *Archiv. Neurol. Psychiatry*, **36**, 1225–1235.

HUTT, S.J., NEWTON, J. and FAIRWEATHER, H. (1977) Choice reaction time and EEG activity in children with epilepsy. *Neuropsychologia*, **15**, 257–267.

ISHIHARA, T. and YOSHII, N. (1967) The interaction between paroxysmal EEG activities and continuous addition work of Uchida–Kraepelin Psychodiagnostic Test. *Med. J. Osaka Univ.*, **18**, 75–85.

KASTELEIJN-NOLST TRENITÉ, D.G.A., RIEMERSMA, J.B.J., BINNIE, C.D., SMIT, A.M. and MEINARDI, H. (1987) The influence of subclinical epileptiform EEG discharges on driving behaviour. *Electroencephal. Clin. Neurophysiol.*, **67**, 167–170.

KASTELEIJN-NOLST TRENITÉ, D.G.A., BAKKER, D.J., BINNIE, C.D., BUERMAN, A. and VAN RAAIJ M. (1988) Psychological effects of sub-clinical epileptiform discharges: Scholastic skills. *Epilepsy Res.* (in press).

RUGLAND, A.L., BJØÆS, H., HENRIKSON, O. and LØYNING, A. (1987). The development of computerized tests as a routine procedure in clinical EEG practice for the evaluation of cognitive changes in patients with epilepsy. *17th Epilepsy International Congress: Abstracts*, p. 102.

SCHWAB R.S. (1939) A method of measuring consciousness in petit mal epilepsy. *J. Nerv. Mental Dis.*, **89**, 690–691.

SIEBELINK, B.M., BAKKER, D.J., BINNIE, C.D. and KASTELEIJN-NOLST TRENITÉ, D.G.A. (1988) Psychological effects of sub-clinical epileptiform EEG discharges in children: General intelligence tests. *Epilepsy Res.* (in press).

5

Seizures, EEG discharges and behaviour

Peter B.C. Fenwick
The Maudsley Hospital, London

INTRODUCTION

A major and significant advance in our understanding of epilepsy occurred in the 1930s with the introduction of the EEG into epilepsy research and clinical practice. It was the recognition that electrical discharges in the EEG correlated with observed seizure behaviour that lead to a taxonomy of epilepsy based on EEG waveforms. Indeed, the first international classification of epilepsy relied heavily on different EEG pictures for different diagnoses. Right from the outset, when the Gibbses were still describing square top waves in temporal lobe epilepsy, there was the realization that scalp potentials were likely to reveal only a fraction of the ongoing cerebral discharges. It was not known, however, whether EEG discharges on the cortex related directly to seizure behaviour or were distinct and separate from those electrical discharges which passed through circuits deep to the cortex, invisible to the surface EEG.

The numerous animal studies made possible by the wider availability of EEG technology after the Second World War demonstrated an imperfect relationship between discharges in the depth and discharges on the surface. However, it was not possible to take advantage of this in man, as the technology for depth electrode use was confined to one or two specialist centres only.

In the 1960s, in the UK, it was standard teaching that an epileptic seizure had to be accompanied by an alteration in cortical rhythms. Alterations in behaviour not accompanied by such changes were thought *not* to be due to epilepsy. This view has been very powerful in shaping attitudes to paroxysmal disorders of behaviour, for it prevented easy acceptance by the orthodox neurological hierarchy of the idea that seizure discharges in the depth could be independent of cortical activity. There were attempts to change this. Such words as epileptoid, epileptic equivalent, etc. which had been employed for

51

many years (Wilson, 1935; Schwab, 1951; Hill, 1981; Reynolds, Chapter 1) were used to describe these disorders of behaviour. However, they failed to gain credibility because there were insufficient data to show that these disorders were caused by true epileptic seizures in the depth and were not due to psychological causes.

NEW WAVE THINKING

Foundation studies

Heath (1986) describes how in the 1950s he embarked on a programme of depth electrode implantation which led him to the recognition that discharges in the amygdala, hippocampus and septal region were at times correlated with paroxysmal changes in behaviour. These results were observed by Monroe (1970) who proposed a specific syndrome, called episodic dyscontrol (Fenwick, 1986, review). This was based on the idea that paroxysmal disorders of behaviour arise from paroxysmal discharges of subcortical structures which were not necessarily recorded in the EEG from the surface of the cortex (Heath and Mickle, 1960; Sem-Jacobson, 1968).

Unfortunately, the concept of episodic dyscontrol has become debased. In its pure form it was considered to be a paroxysmal disorder of behaviour arising from limbic discharges in patients with a normal personality. However, the term came to include other disorders of behaviour such as disorders of personality, or disorders due to brain damage or social factors, which were not solely due to abnormal limbic discharges. (For a review see Fenwick, 1986a.)

In the mid-1970s many different units started to implant depth electrodes as part of the work-up for patients who were to undergo temporal lobectomy. This work enabled the occurrence of paroxysmal seizure discharges in the depth, involving limbic structures, the amygdala and hippocampus, without spread to the cortex to be established (Mark and Ervin, 1970; Hitchcock and Cairns, 1973; Wieser, 1983a).

Any unit that carries out depth recordings now accepts that seizure discharges within the depth do not necessarily have to propagate to the surface, and that *some* of these limbic discharges *may* be accompanied by changes in behaviour. A recent example is shown in Fig. 1. This is taken from the work of Wieser (1983a) and it shows the presence of high voltage seizure discharges within the limbic structures producing aggressive behaviour, but not affecting cortical rhythms to any degree. Wieser comments: 'Prior to SEEG exploration these rage attacks were not believed to be of epileptic origin, and the patient was mistakenly diagnosed as an "aggressive psychopath". . . . The neurological examination showed a left tempero-basal cyst communicating with the temporal horn . . .' Removal of the cyst resulted in a marked improvement of the epilepsy and the aggressive behaviour.

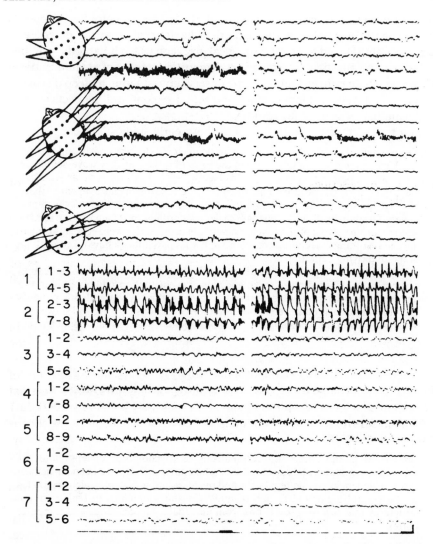

Fig. 1 Depth recorded limbic seizures. During a rage attack a long-lasting clonic discharge in the left periamygdalar region was recorded (1 and 2). Two sections at the beginning of the second and fourth minute of this seizure are shown. Calibration: 1 sec, 50 V, TC 0.3, F = 70. Reprinted with permission from *Neuroscience and Behavioural Reviews*, **7**, 427–40, Wieser, H.G., 1983, Pergamon Journals Ltd.

In the 1950s and 1960s Heath (1986) was studying discharges from the limbic system with implanted electrodes, not only in patients with epilepsy but also in patients who did not have clinical seizures and were diagnosed as suffering from schizophrenia. He reported that these patients also showed epileptiform activity in the form of spikes. He noted a relationship between this spiking in the depth and hallucinatory experiences. At that time the diagnosis of schizophrenia lacked the methodological precision which it has today, so there must be some question as to the exact diagnostic category of Heath's patients. However, there is little doubt that the observations relating to deep discharges within the amygdala, hippocampus and septal regions and the occurrence of hallucinatory behaviour are valid.

In a recent review, Heath describes those early studies:

> The psychotic behaviour of patients with deep electrodes was consistently corre-
> lated with a recording abnormality in the form of spike and slow wave activity in
> the rostral-septal region (Heath 1954, Heath 1975). In those patients who had
> electrodes in the lateral amygdala, the recording abnormality also appeared there
> . . . but the significant correlation was with the abnormal activity in the septal
> region. Despite the dramatic changes in deep recordings, no changes were seen in
> scalp recording. Most of the psychotic patients in our series were schizophrenics,
> but the recording correlation was consistent with psychotic behaviour regardless
> of its underlying aetiology . . .
>
> During interictal periods, numerous epileptic patients without complicating
> psychotic behaviour showed spike and slow wave activity predominantly in the
> hippocampus with no involvement of the septal region. A few epileptic patients
> had episodes of psychotic behaviour. On those occasions, spiking and slow wave
> activity appeared in recordings of the septal region as well as the hippocampus.
> (Figure 2.) (Review and quote from Heath, 1986; Heath and Walker, 1985;
> Heath, 1962).

The demonstration by Heath of spike activity in the septum correlating with hallucinatory behaviour has given rise to the speculation that these structures may be involved in schizophrenia, and that deep spike foci may be part of the pathology of schizophrenia. This model of schizophrenia has been extended by Stevens who noted

> similarities in the auras and automatisms of psychomotor epilepsy and the
> subjective symptoms and stereotypes of schizophrenia. We have been particular-
> ly interested in dopamine regulation and the mesolimbic system, which originates
> in the ventral tegmental nucleii of midbrain and terminates in limbic striatal
> structures that receive projections from amygdala, hippocampus and temporal
> cortex . . .

Stimulation by a reduction of inhibitory feedback in the ventral-tegmental area in waking, unrestrained cats, produced

> behavioural states of hypervigilance, searching, hiding, fear, and repeated orien-
> tating activity, during which spikes are recorded from the ipsilateral nucleus
> accumbens, essentially the same region from which Heath recorded spike activity
> in schizophrenic man (Stevens et al., 1974). Similarly spike activity and changed
> behaviour were also induced after kindling of ventral tegmental area (in cats).
> (Stevens, 1977)

Whether or not spike activity of itself is necessarily pathological has been questioned by many authors. There is certainly evidence that spikes are found in the EEG in many non-epileptic conditions, for example sleep, depressive

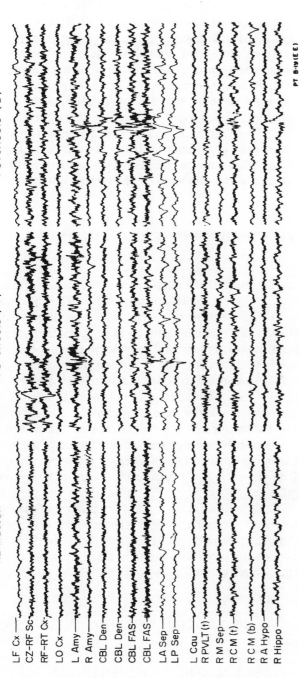

Fig. 2 Recordings from a schizophrenic patient when his symptoms had remitted and when he was psychotic.

Abbreviations: AMY = amygdala, CAU = caudate nucleus, CM = centro median thalamus, CX = cortex, CZ = central zero scalp, DEN = dentate nucleus, FAS = fastial nucleus of the cerebellum, GENIC = geniculate, HIP = hippocampus, HYP = hypothalamus, L = left, M = medial, OCC = occipital, PALL = pallidum, PAR = parietal, PVL = posterior ventral lateral, R = right, SEP = septal region, SUP = superior, TEMP = temporal, THAL = thalamus.

illnesses, childhood, etc. Thus the nature of spikes recorded from limbic structures in hallucinating man may not necessarily be pathological, but may be part of normal function. So the occurrence of spike activity in the depth, in the absence of a clear epileptic condition, should be interpreted with caution. However, what have been clearly established are three fundamental principles. First, that epileptic activity in the depth need not necessarily be accompanied by changes in scalp activity; secondly, that these discharges may be accompanied by paroxysmal changes in behaviour; and thirdly, that epileptic (-like?) discharges in the limbic system can be associated with abnormal mental states. Perhaps new methods of brain exploration and imaging could help. The infant science of magneto-encephalography, which has the potential to visualize deep coherent magnetic sources within the brain, is one such possibility (Fenwick, 1987).

DEPTH ELECTRODES AND SEIZURE DISCHARGES

There is a burgeoning literature on the relationship between seizure discharges deep within the brain and their clinical manifestations. This information is obtained from patients who are being prepared for epilepsy surgery, and thus suffers from the disadvantage that most patients have severe and unremitting epilepsy, or significant associated cerebral pathology. Despite these limitations, it is now possible to trace the origin of seizures deep to the superficial layers of the cortex, their spread to nearby cerebral structures and the form that the clinical seizures may take. These new data raise several important questions relating to our understanding of seizure types and the likely diagnostic information that can be obtained by the observation of seizure behaviour. What is now clear is that seizures arising in very different parts of the brain may give rise to almost identical clinical signs. This raises the important question whether the classification of seizures by their clinical features is any longer an appropriate method, especially in research studies which set out to look at cognitive function. Seizures arising in different brain structures were expected to produce different focal cognitive deficits. There is also an increasing literature on the relationship between scalp EEG activity and seizure origin. In many cases these two are not congruent and thus it is difficult to be sure that focal scalp discharges are a true indication of seizure onset.

TEMPORAL LOBE EPILEPSY

There are now approximately 50 centres throughout the world which carry out epilepsy surgery. Many of these implant depth electrodes. The method of

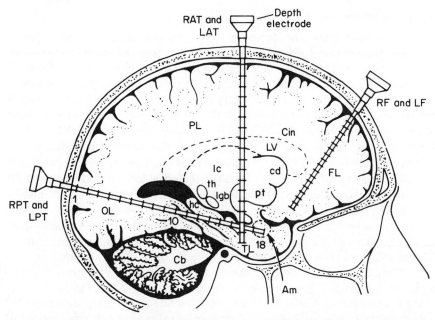

Fig. 3   Common array of electrodes for frontal and temporal lobe studies. RAT and LAT = electrodes inserted through frontal lobe structures into the temporal lobes, RF and LF = frontal lobe electrodes, RPT and LPT = occipital insertion studying the length of the hippocampus, OL = occipital lobe, PL = parietal lobe, Cin = cingulate gyrus, FL = frontal lobe, LV = lateral ventricle, cd = caudate, lc = internal capsule, th = thalamus, pt = putamen, Am = amygdala. Reproduced from Engel, J. (ed.) (1987) *Surgical Treatment of the Epilepsies*. p. 683, by permission of Raven Press, New York.

implantation varies from unit to unit. For an excellent review of the different methods used see Engel (1987). Most centres use multi-contact electrodes with spacings of a few millimetres which can allow accurate location of seizure onset (Fig. 3). The brain is, however, very large, and it is possible for electrode placement to miss the site of seizure onset, particularly from the frontal lobes.

However, considerable information is now available on the relationship between seizures which arise in the depth, their subsequent spread through the cortex, and the changes that are produced on the scalp. What this work has shown us is that many of our old concepts relating to the onset and transmission of seizures need revision. It is now clear that our understanding of seizure spread as shown by the scalp EEG is different from the picture provided by depth electrodes. The new information from the depth suggests there is much less specificity in the auras evoked by seizures and in seizure types than was originally thought, as is shown in the following short review. A more comprehensive and fuller review is given by Williamson et al. (1987).

Temporal lobe seizures

Seizures arising from the temporal lobe are commonly complex partial seizures. Hauser and Kurland (1975) have suggested that between 20% and 40% of all seizure types are complex partial seizures, while a figure of between 70% and 80% of complex partial seizures arising within the temporal lobe is suggested by the temporal lobe surgery groups at Yale and UCLA. Complex partial seizures do not only arise from the temporal lobe, but may arise from other parts of the brain, although this is not always emphasized (O'Donohoe, 1985). Indeed, the frontal lobes are a common source of complex partial seizures (see below). EEG scalp recordings of seizures are only successful in detecting the true site of origin within the temporal lobe in under 50% of the cases reported from units that use depth electrodes. Adding the information provided by sphenoidal electrodes, Rasmussen (1983) estimates that only 60% of attacks can be correctly localized. The studies show that 25% of attacks show a bilateral symmetrical suppression of activity or a generalized onset, and a further 15% add no useful information because the EEG is obscured by artefacts. Thus, in about 33% of cases, in order to be certain that the seizure is arising from one temporal region, it may be necessary to implant depth electrodes.

Studies carried out by units with a temporal lobe surgery programme involve only patients with longstanding and drug resistant epilepsy. It is important to stress that the figures quoted in such studies possibly give an overestimate of the difficulty of seizure location. What these studies do show is that in over a third of cases, scalp localization of both ictal and interictal activity is likely to be inaccurate. This is of particular significance to those research studies which have to locate seizure onset in one or other temporal lobe using only scalp EEG data.

Much of the old teaching concerning experiences during the aura of temporal lobe seizures suggested that seizures which arose from the lateral surface of the temporal lobe were most likely to be associated with complex hallucinations, illusions and memories. A recent study from Montreal suggests that this teaching is wrong, and that the hippocampus and amygdala are not only involved but crucial to the genesis of hallucinations, illusions and memories (see Figure 4, Gloor, 1986). The Paris and Montreal groups have reported that olfactory hallucinations arise from seizures commencing in the uncus, elementary auditory hallucinations from Heschl's gyrus, vertiginous sensations from posterior temporal operculum, and gustatory symptoms from the insula.

Delgado-Escueta et al. (1981) studied 691 seizures in 79 patients using video monitoring and defined classical forms of temporal lobe seizures. They were able to define two distinct types, which they called Type I and Type II. Type I was thought to arise from mesial temporal structures, and was characterized by:

(a) arrest reactions or motionless stare. At first the patient is unresponsive to stimuli. Sometimes the attack may start with déjà vu feelings, or abdominal, olfactory or gustatory perceptions.

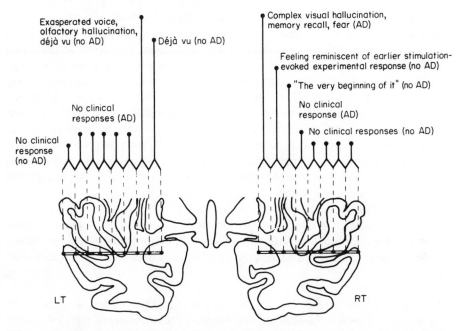

Exasperated voice, olfactory hallucination, déjà vu (no AD)

Déjà vu (no AD)

Complex visual hallucination, memory recall, fear (AD)

Feeling reminiscent of earlier stimulation-evoked experimental response (no AD)

"The very beginning of it" (no AD)

No clinical responses (AD)

No clinical response (AD)

No clinical responses (no AD)

No clinical response (no AD)

LT

RT

Fig. 4   Topographical distribution of responses obtained in one patient with electrical stimulations applied to adjacent pairs of contacts 5 mm apart along two horizontal depth electrode trajectories through the left and right temporal lobes. Electrode contacts 1 and 2 (most mesial) are within the amygdala; most of the others are in contact with temporal neocortical grey matter. The height of the vertical lines roughly indicates the intensity of responses elicited by electrical stimulations. AD = afterdischarge, LT = left, RT = right. Reproduced from Gloor, P. (1986) In: Doane, B.K. and Livingstone, K.E. (eds) *The Limbic System: Functional Organization and Clinical Disorders*. By permission of Raven Press, New York.

(b) stereotyped, automatic, oro-alimentary behaviour such as chewing, swallowing or lip-smacking.
(c) severely impaired consciousness.
(d) automatisms, with gradual recovery and the automatisms becoming more complex and responsive to the environment.

Type II seizures were distinguished from Type I in that there was no initial motionless stare, the seizures beginning with semi-purposeful motor activity. These were initially thought to arise from the lateral surface of the temporal lobe, but later Delgado-Escueta thought they could be extra-temporal, possibly frontal (Walsh and Delgado-Escueta, 1984).

It is now clear that the above scheme is over simplified. Recent data from depth implanted electrodes (Maldonado et al., 1986) in the medial temporal structures, suggest that only 30% of seizures start with a motionless stare, 26% have an onset of simple automatisms, but in 40% there is a more complex onset which is similar to lateral temporal or extra-temporal seizures. This gives a very different view of the accuracy of localizing seizure onset, and stresses how difficult it is to localize the onset of a seizure using behavioural changes. Williamson (1986) reported on depth electrode data derived from the operative series at Yale. The Yale descriptions of Type I seizures do not differ from those of Moldonado et al. They list an unobtrusive onset, usually characterized by an arrest, or simple stereotyped automatisms, including vocalization, with progress to more complex automatisms. Tonic postures were common. There was progressive post ictal recovery. The Paris group suggest that oro-alimentary automatisms arise from the amygdala. Complex automatisms are thought by both the Paris and Montreal groups to be bilateral hippocampal and to have little localizing value.

Wieser (1983b) in a comprehensive statistical study, derived from the electro-clinical data of detailed depth electrode investigation in patients being prepared for temporal lobe surgery, defined four major forms of temporal lobe seizure onset. These could be differentiated by the use of discriminant function analysis.

1. *Tempero-basal limbic*. This was the most frequent type. There were auras of déjà vu, memory flashbacks, and epigastric sensations, in 80% of cases. Consciousness was maintained as long as the seizure remained unilateral. Later in the seizure there was sudden arresting or a motionless stare, but these signs were not specific to this seizure type. Although oro-alimentary automatisms were common, they did not arise early in the seizure. Complex automatisms were seen after the discharge had spread bilaterally. Unilateral or bilateral tonic or tonic-clonic activity was common.
2. *Temporal polar seizures*. These were similar to temporo-basal limbic but had prominent early autonomic changes and early oro-alimentary automatisms.
3. *Opercular seizures* were characterized by auditory hallucinations, which arose from seizure spread to Heschl's gyrus. There was focal motor activity, especially in the face and upper extremities. Aphasia occurred rarely, and apparently could occur with seizure onset in either the dominant or non-dominant hemisphere.
4. *Posterior temporal neo-cortical*. These exhibited vestibular auras and complex visual hallucinations. Because of rapid spread, only the first 10–30 seconds is useful for identifying the region of onset.

Overview of temporal lobe seizures

A summary of seizure types is given by Williamson et al. (1987). They report that certain common characteristics can be detected in temporal lobe seizures arising from the mesial structures. These are the Type 1 seizures of Delgado-

Escueta, the medio-basal limbic seizures of Wieser, and the primarily rhinencephalic seizures of Bancaud. Over 80% of TLE seizures begin in the mesial structures. Between 70 and 90% of patients have auras, but they tend to be non-specific, and are often accompanied by early non-specific autonomic activity. The arrest reaction is not specific and may be related to seizure spread. Initial automatisms are usually simple. Complex automatisms tend to follow the ictus and tonic motor activity is common. Motor activity may result from extra temporal spread and there is some suggestion that the cingulate gyrus may become involved. There is usually a definite change from ictal to post ictal state with a gradual return to awareness after the seizure.

FRONTAL LOBE SEIZURES

Exploration of the frontal lobes is difficult because of their sheer size. Bancaud et al. (1965) frequently stressed how difficult it is to locate accurately the onset of frontal lobe seizures, and several exploratory implantations of electrodes may be necessary. Frontal lobe seizures are so varied in type that no clear frontal lobe syndrome has as yet been described. Petit mal, generalized, partial, or partial-complex seizures have all been described as arising from the frontal lobes. Seizures with a focal onset are known to spread rapidly and become generalized. Thus their focal onset may be obscured by the rapid spread. Although there is now more understanding that partial complex seizures do not only arise in the temporal lobes, many frontal lobe seizures which are partial complex in character may still be missed.

Rolandic seizures

Depth electrodes have contributed little to our already extensive understanding of seizures arising in the Rolandic area. Classical Jacksonian marches and seizures with precise localization indicated by tonic-clonic features are well known. Epilepsia partialis continuans or focal status of the motor cortex has been reported by depth electrodes (Wieser et al., 1978; Wieser, 1983c).

Seizures in the supplementary motor area

Tonic postures are part of the usual clinical expression of supplementary motor seizures. Typically, they consist of head and eyes deviated to the opposite side, with abduction and external rotation of the opposite arm, with flexion of the elbow. Although this posture of the patient looking at his own hand is thought to be specific, it is often seen in association with leg extension, elevation or flexion. Until secondary generalization occurs, consciousness is usually retained. There have been several reports in the literature which suggest that the stereotyped posture already described is an oversimplification of the various forms of tonic posturing which can occur. Other authors have noted that typical Rolandic posturing may occur either from other brain areas or because seizures have spread to the pre-Rolandic region (Ajmone-Marsan and Ralston, 1957; Bancaud et al., 1965; Niedermeyer, 1974; Wieser, 1983c).

An interesting group of seizures attributed to this area by Niedermeyer (1974) are brief, frequent seizures without interictal or ictal EEG abnormalities which begin and end suddenly. They are frequently precipitated by a startle. These, Niedermeyer suggests, are mesio-frontal, and possibly spread into the pre-Rolandic area.

Orbital frontal seizures

These are of considerable interest because they commence with prominent autonomic activity, with or without head deviation. Indeed, there have been suggestions in the literature that this type of frontal seizure cannot be distinguished from seizures that originate in the temporal lobes. Tharp (1972) has postulated a specific orbito-frontal syndrome. This commenced with noticeable autonomic changes, loud noises and walking movements, followed by automatisms. EEG sharp activity was commonly seen in the interictal EEG. This syndrome was based on only three cases, and other authors have had less success in finding it. Indeed, Ludwig et al. (1975) looking at a group of patients with seizures of probable orbital frontal origin stressed autonomic activity with or without head and eye deviation, often followed by generalization.

Dorso-lateral frontal seizures and frontal polar seizures

Seizures starting in these areas generalize rapidly, often without any clear clinical evidence of a focal onset. The clinical features of the seizures are usually due to posterior spread into the pre-Rolandic area. There is a suggestion by Delgado-Escueta (1986) that brief tonic and absence like seizures may arise from the dorso-frontal region. Adversive seizures with early unconsciousness arising in the frontal polar regions are distinguished on clinical grounds from adversive seizures with maintained consciousness which arise from the pre-Rolandic area (Gastaut, 1954; Ajmone-Marsan and Ralston, 1957).

Frontal lobe complex partial seizures

For many years it has been recognized that complex partial seizures are not specifically temporal but can arise from many different brain areas, the most important of which are the frontal lobes. Penfield and Christiansen (1951) suggested that frontal automatisms are different from those of the temporal lobe in that they had a pseudo-voluntary nature. Seizures arising in nearly every frontal area have been described, commencing with either a psychical aura or limited motor automatisms, progressing to more complex automatisms with semi-purposeful motor activity as consciousness is regained. A recent paper from the Yale group (Williamson et al., 1985a), using implanted depth electrodes, has suggested that there is a specific syndrome of frontal lobe partial seizures. They have suggested that there are brief seizures lasting up to about 30 seconds, with a sudden beginning and ending, and minimal post ictal confusion. Prominent, complex, semi-purposeful motor automatisms which may include sexual automatisms, are common. Forced vocalization occurs and the patients often report non-specific auras. What is of interest is that many of these complex automatisms are bizarre, and frequently patients may be referred from the psychiatric services because they have previously been diagnosed as suffering from hysteria. The attacks tend to be stereotyped for each individual patient, and they occur in clusters of several per day. Of considerable interest is the occurrence of complex partial status in this group of patients, also explored by the Yale group with depth electrodes (Williamson et al., 1985b). Swartz and Delgardo-Escueta (1987) are less certain that frontal complex partial status can easily be recognized owing to its rapid spread. This again shows the importance of depth recording.

Generalized seizures originating in the frontal lobe

An exploration of the literature relating to seizures arising in the frontal lobe soon convinces the reader that frontal lobe generalized seizures are very common. Indeed, as both generalized seizures and petit mal seizures can originate from the frontal lobes, the old concept of primary generalized epilepsy must be called more and more into question. The advent of CT scans and MRI scans has now significantly reduced the population of patients with epilepsy but without any apparent brain lesion. Presumably, subtler forms of brain investigation could uncover yet smaller lesions in those cases that are still considered to be idiopathic. The frontal lobes are certainly likely to be intimately involved with the genesis of many or most of the generalized seizures. Bancaud (1969) showed that seizures arising from the mesial frontal region could be generalized from the start, and he also described how stimulation of the mesial frontal cortex resulted in typical petit mal and grand mal attacks. Goldring (1972) noted that many generalized seizures originated in the prefrontal cortex. Also, no clinical signs suggestive of a focal onset can be seen in seizures originating in the lateral frontal cortex (Niedermeyer, 1974).

Overview of frontal lobe seizures

In summary, motor features are common and prominent in front lobe seizures. Focal features at the onset, apart from those arising in the Rolandic and pre-Rolandic regions, may be brief and easily missed, as the seizures tend to generalize rapidly. Auras are common but not specific. Both generalized convulsive status and partial complex status occur. Highly complex motor activity of a pseudo-voluntary nature may occur, leading to the diagnosis of hysteria. This should be borne in mind by the psychiatric clinician with an interest in epilepsy. The physician should be cautious about changing the drug regime of frontal lobe patients too rapidly, because of the ease with which status epilepticus may occur.

CONCLUSION

Depth electrode studies have revolutionized our understanding of the brain. They have shown us that many of the earlier concepts about precise clinical symptoms following epileptic discharges in specific brain areas are incorrect. The brain responds in a much more variable fashion and seizures arising in a specific brain area may track in different directions and lead to completely different clinical pictures. Thus, the original specificity attributed to auras must now be reconsidered. Although complex partial seizures probably arise mainly in the temporal lobe, they can occur in many other brain areas, the frontal lobes being the most common.

Depth electrode studies have shown convincingly that seizures within the depth may lead to paroxysmal disorders of behaviour with no spread of seizure activity from the limbic structures to the cortex. The significance of this observation has yet to become apparent to many practising neurologists and psychiatrists. For as Monroe initially postulated, many paroxysmal disorders of behaviour can now again be attributed to abnormal cerebral functioning. Clearly, further non-invasive methods for detecting abnormal discharges within the depth are now required. Brain imaging using metabolic measures such as PET and SPECT may give some information on areas of abnormal metabolism in the depth and this may correlate either positively or negatively with deep epileptic discharges. The infant science of magnetoencephalography may yet be able, by locating coherent magnetic sources within the depth, to contribute information concerning the precise nature and location of these deep discharging foci. The next few years can be expected to see a rapprochement of neurology and psychiatry as both turn to recognize the true importance of abnormal discharges within the depth of the brain.

REFERENCES

AJMONE-MARSAN, C. and RALSTON, B.L. (1957) *The Epileptic Seizure. Its functional morphology and diagnostic significance.* Charles C. Thomas, Springfield, Illinois.

BANCAUD, J. (1969) Physiopathogenesis of generalised epilepsies of organic nature (stereo-electro-encepahlographic study). In *Physiopathogenesis of the Epilepsies* (ed. H. GASTAUT), pp. 158–185. Charles C. Thomas, Springfield, Illinois.

BANCAUD, J., TALAIRACH, J., BONIS, A., SCHAUB, A., SZIKALA, G., MOREL, P. and BORDAS-FERRER, M. (1965) *La Stéréo-electroencephalographie dans L'épilepsie.* Masson, Paris.

DELGADO-ESCUETA, A., BACSAL, F. and TREIMAN, D. (1981). Complex partial seizures on close circuit television and EEG: a study of 691 attacks in 79 patients. *Ann. Neurol.*, **11**, 292–300.

DELGADO-ESCUETA, A.V., Swartz, B. MALDONADO, H., WALSH, G., RAND, R. and HALGREN, E. (1986) Complex partial seizures of frontal lobe origin. In *Pre-surgical Evaluation of Epileptics* (ed. WIESER, H. and ELGER, C.). Springer, Heidelberg.

ENGEL, J. (ed.) (1987) *Surgical Treatment of the Epilepsies.* pp. 583–635. Raven Press. New York.

FENWICK, P.B.C. (1986a) Is dyscontrol epilepsy? In REYNOLDS, E.H. and TRIMBLE, M. (eds) *What is Epilepsy?* Churchill-Livingstone, Edinburgh.

FENWICK, P.B.C. (1986b) Aggression and epilepsy. In TRIMBLE, M. and BOLWIG, T. (eds) *Aspects of Epilepsy and Psychiatry.* John Wiley & Sons, Chichester.

FENWICK, P.B.C. (1987) The inverse problem — a medical perspective. *Phys. Med. Biol.*, **32**, pp. 5–9.

GASTAUT, H. (1954) *The Epilepsies, Electro-clinical Correlations.* Charles C. Thomas, Springfield, Illinois.

GLOOR, P. (1986) Role of the human limbic system in perception, memory, and affect: lessons from temporal lobe epilepsy. In *The Limbic System: Functional Organisation and Clinical Disorders.* (eds. B. DOANE, and K. LIVINGSTONE). Raven Press. New York.

GOLDRING, S. (1972) The role of prefrontal cortex in grand mal convulsion. *Arch. Neurol.*, **26**, 109–119.

HAUSER, W. and KURLAND, L. (1975) The epidemiology of epilepsy in Rochester, Minnesota, 1935 through 1967. *Epilepsia*, **16**, 1–66.

HEATH, R.G. (1954) Tulane University Department of Psychiatry and Neurology. *Studies in Schizophrenia.* Harvard University Press, Cambridge, Mass.

HEATH, R.G. (1962) Common characteristics of epilepsy and schizophrenia: clinical observations and depth electrode studies. *Am. J Psychiat.*, **188**, 1013–1026.

Heath, R.G. (1975) Brain function and behaviour: emotional and sensory phenomena in psychotic patients and in experimental animals. *J. Nerv. Ment. Dis.*, **160**, 159–175.

HEATH, R.G. (1986) Studies with deep electrodes in patients intractably ill with epilepsy and other disorders. In REYNOLDS, E. and TRIMBLE, M. (eds) *What is Epilepsy?* Churchill-Livingstone, Edinburgh.

HEATH, R.G. and MICKLE, W.A. (1960) Evaluation of seven years experience with depth electrode studies in human patients. In RAMEY, E.R., O'DOHERTY, D. (eds) *Electrical Studies of the Unanaesthetised Brain.* pp. 214–247. Paul, B. Hober, New York.

HEATH, R.G. and WALKER, C.F. (1985) Correlations of deep and surface electroencephalograms with psychosis and hallucinations in schizophrenics: a report of two cases. *Biol. Psychiat.*, **20**, 669–674.

HILL, D. (1981) Historical review. *Epilepsy and Psychiatry* (eds REYNOLDS, E.H. and TRIMBLE, M.). Churchill-Livingstone. Edinburgh.

HITCHCOCK, E. and CAIRNS, V. (1973) Amygdalotomy. *Postgrad. Med. J.*, **49**, 894–904.

LUDWIG, B., AJMONE-MARSAN, C. and VAN BUREN, J. (1975) Cerebral seizures of probable orbito-frontal origin. *Epilepsia*, **16**, 141–158.

MALDONADO, H.M. DELGADO-ESCUETA, A., RAND, R., WALSH, G., HALGREN, E., TREIMAN, D. and BERMAN, D. (1986) Complex partial seizures of hippocampal and amygdalal origin: 1. Electrobehavioural features. *Annals of Neurology* (in press). Reported in *Surgical Treatment of the Epilepsies* (ed. ENGEL, J.). Raven Press, p. 102, (1987).

MARK, V.H. and ERVIN, F. (1970) *Violence and the Brain.* Harper and Row, New York.

MAZARS, G. (1969) Cingulate gyrus epileptogenic foci as an origin for generalised seizures. In *The Physiopathogenesis of the Epilepsies* (eds GASTAUT, H., JASPER, H.,

BANCAUD, J. and WALTREGNY, A.), pp. 186–189. Charles C. Thomas, Springfield, Illinois.

MONROE, R. (1970) *Episodic Behavioural Disorders*. Harvard University Press, Cambridge, Mass.

NIEDERMEYER, E. (1974) *Compendium of the Epilepsies*. Charles C. Thomas, Springfield, Illinois.

O'DONAHOE, O.V. (1985) Partial seizures of complex symptomatology (temporal lobe epilepsy). In *Epilepsies of Childhood*, 2nd edition, pp. 92–105. Butterworths, London.

PENFIELD, W., and CRISTIANSEN, K. (1951) *Epileptic Seizure Patterns*. Charles C. Thomas, Springfield, Illinois.

RASMUSSEN, T.B. (1983) Surgical treatment of complex partial seizures: results, lessons, and problems, *Epilepsia*, **24** (Suppl. 1), S65–76.

SCHWAB, R.S. (1951) *Electroencephalography*. W.B. Saunders, London.

SEM-JACOBSON, C.W. (1968) Vegetative changes in response to electrical brain stimulation. *Electroenceph. Clin. Neurophysiol.*, **24**, 28.

STEVENS, J. (1977) All that spikes is not fits. In *Psychopathology and Brain Dysfunction* pp. 183–198 (eds GERSHON, S. and FRIEDHOF, A.). Raven Press. New York. Reprinted in *What is Epilepsy?* pp. 97–109 (eds TRIMBLE M. and REYNOLDS, E.H., 1986). Churchill-Livingstone, Edinburgh.

STEVENS, J., WILSON, K. and FOOTE, W. (1974) GABA blockade, dopamine and schizophrenia. Experimental studies in the cat. *Psychopharmacologia*, **39**, 105–119.

STOFFELS, C. et al. (1981) Seizures of the anterior cingulate gyrus in man. A stereo-EEG study, *Proc. of Epilepsy International Symposium Kyoto*, pp. 85–86. Raven Press. New York.

SWARTZ, B.E. and DELGADO-ESCUETA, A.V. (1987) The management of status epilepticus. In *Epilepsy* (ed. HOPKINS, A.), p. 422. Chapman and Hall, London.

THARP, B.R. (1972) Orbital frontal seizures. A unique electroencephalographic and clinical syndrome, *Epilepsia*, **13**, 627–642.

WALSH, G. and DELGADO-ESCUETA, A. (1984) Type 2 complex partial seizures: poor results from anterior temporal lobectomy. *Neurology*, **34**, 1–13.

WIESER, H.G. (1983a) Depth recorded limbic seizures and psychopathology. *Neuroscience and Behavioural Review*, **7** (3), 427–440.

WIESER, H.G. (1983b). *Electroclinical Features of the Psychomotor Seizure*. Gustav Fischer, Stuttgart.

WIESER, H. (1983c) Stereoelectroencephalographic correlates of focal motor seizures. In *Epilepsia and Motor System* (eds SPECKMAN, E. and ELGER, C.), pp. 287–309. Urban and Schwarzenberg. Munich.

WIESER, H., GRAF, H., BERNOULLI, C. and SIEGFRIED, J. (1978) Quantitive analysis of intracerebral recordings in epilepsia partialis continua. *Electroenceph. Clin. Neurophysiol.*, **44**, 14–22.

WILLIAMSON, P.D. (1986) Intensive monitoring for complex partial seizures. In *Advances in Neurology* (ed. GUMNIT, R.). Raven Press. New York.

WILLIAMSON, P.D., SPENCER, D., SPENCER, S., NOVELLI, R. and MATTSON, R. (1985a) Complex partial seizures of frontal lobe origin. *Ann. Neurol.*, **18**, 497–504.

WILLIAMSON, P.D., SPENCER, S., MATTSON, R. and SPENCER, D. (1985b) Complex partial status epilepticus. A depth electrode study. *Ann. Neurol.*, **18**, 647–654.

WILLIAMSON, P.D. WIESER, H.G. and DELGADO-ESCUETA, A. (1987) Clinical characteristics of partial seizures. *Surgical Treatments of the Epilepsies* (ed. ENGEL, J.). Raven Press. New York.

WILSON, S.A. KINNIE (1935) *The Epilepsies. Handbuch der Neurologie*, **IX**. Springer, Berlin, pp. 1–84.

6

Anticonvulsants, seizures and performance: The Veteran's Administration experience*

Dennis B. Smith
Comprehensive Epilepsy Program of Oregon, Good Samaritan Hospital and Medical Center, Portland, Oregon, USA

INTRODUCTION

Until very recently, it has been difficult to tease out specific behavioural or cognitive effects of individual AEDs. Global improvement or even improvement in specific areas of function when polypharmacy is rationalized allows the inference that the previous deficits were caused by the drug removed. It is a reasonable inference, but it is possible that the deficits attributed to specific drugs were in fact caused by adverse drug interactions or even the addition of similar toxicities, and that the improvement was due in part to better patient management. Administering single AEDs to normal volunteers has provided significant information about the toxicities of individual AEDs but for ethical reasons, assessment of long-term behavioural effects of these drugs by this method is not practical. Similarly, crossover studies, when one drug used as monotherapy is replaced by another drug also used as monotherapy, present an ethical dilemma if seizure control has been achieved on the first drug; and a statistical dilemma if a substantial difference in seizure frequency develops between the treatment groups.

In 1985, a nationwide multicentre comparison of the efficacy and toxicity of carbamazepine (CBZ), phenobarbital (Pb), phenytoin (PHT), and primidone (PRM) was completed (Mattson et al., 1985). The study was a five-year double-blind prospective trial conducted by the Veterans Administration involving ten

* This work was supported by a V.A. Cooperative Studies (No.118) Grant.

Veteran Administration Medical Centers across the country. Analysis of neuropsychological data obtained during that study is providing important new insights into specific cognitive and behavioural effects of different AEDs, but also the effects of epilepsy itself. The large number of patients entered into the study as well as the careful study design has provided a unique opportunity to examine the behavioural characteristics of patients with epilepsy who are unaffected by AEDs and to compare these characteristics with normal controls matched for age, sex and educational level. The ability to use each patient as their own control and to examine behavioural change over a prolonged period of time while on monotherapy are other important features of this study. This chapter summarizes some of the results of that study.

METHODS

Study design

Six hundred and twenty-two patients with well-documented simple or complex partial seizures, or primary or secondarily generalized tonic-clonic seizures, who were newly diagnosed and drug naive, or who were undertreated, were enrolled in the study. Three hundred and fifty-five patients were classified as having secondary generalized tonic-clonic seizures, 222 with primarily partial

Table 1.   Exclusions

1. Under age 18
2. Diagnosis of epilepsy not confirmed
3. Classification of specific seizure type not possible
4. Aetiology of seizure is neoplastic, progressive degenerative, metabolic, demyelinateing, or active infection (a patient with a previously resected tumour that is not recurrent is acceptable)
5. Patient has generalized seizures but not tonic-clinic (e.g. only absence)
6. Abuse of alcohol ($\geq$ four drinks per day)
7. Abuse of other drugs (e.g. narcotics)
8. Patient has progressive neurological disorder
9. Patient has serious medical disorder (unstable or requiring intervention or both) or active infection
10. Patient is psychotic, grossly organic or severely depressed
11. Patient's intelligence quotient (WAIS) full-scale is less than 85
12. Patient is a wilful noncomplier
13. Repeated seizures may occur under a variety of circumstances related to acute medical disorders such as uremia, hypoglycemia, etc., and are not considered epilepsy for the purpose of this study

complex seizures, and 61 as having partial simple seizures. The mean age of seizure onset was 29.8 years. A mean of 12.2 years had elapsed between the first seizure and enrolment in the study. Many of these patients had never sought treatment despite this interval, and none had received more than intermittent treatment. Details of entry criteria and design have been reported elsewhere (Delgado-Escueta et al., 1983; Mattson, 1983; Cramer et al., 1983). Table 1 lists the strict exclusion criteria used in the study, and emphasizes the care used to ensure that the study population closely matched a typical out-patient population.

After careful classification by predominant seizure type, patients were randomized to one of the four study drugs (CBZ, PHT, Pb, or PRM). The dose of each drug was then increased until 'mid' to 'high' therapeutic range had been achieved. If seizure control was not adequate, the dose was then pushed further until intolerable toxicity was produced and then reduced. The blinded investigator had no knowledge of the antiepileptic drug level when adjusting dose and relied on the unblinded monitor. Whenever possible, the dosage was increased to the point of clinical toxicity and then backed off *even* if seizure control had apparently been achieved. The goal was to reassess the published therapeutic ranges for each of the four AEDs.

Neuropsychological tests

Again, whenever possible a full battery of neuropsychological tests was performed on each patient before the patient was randomized to one of the four study drugs. This same battery was then repeated at one month, three months, and every six months thereafter. Seventy-five control subjects matched closely for age, sex and education were administered the same battery of neuropsychological tests on two occasions, one month apart. The tests have been well described and are part of the Halsted–Reitan Neuropsychological Test Battery or the Lafayette Repeatable Neuropsychological Battery (Lewis, 1979). These behavioural methods have been shown by others (Reitan and Davidson, 1974; Lewis and Rennick, 1979; Dodrill, 1981) to be sensitive indicators of subtle cognitive dysfunction that may be associated with AED use. The specific tests used in this battery were selected in order to reflect neuropsychological functioning in four major areas:

1. general intellect
2. attention/concentration/mental flexibility
3. motor/motor manipulation
4. emotional/mood states.

General intellectual ability was measured by the Weschler Adult Intelligence Scale (WAIS), a well-standardized measure of general cognitive function based on eleven verbal and nonverbal subtest activities. Attention/

concentration was measured using digit symbol substitution, digit span, critical flicker fusion, discriminative reaction time, and word finding. Motor and motor manipulative functions are reflected in index finger tapping, Lafayette pegboard and colour naming. Colour naming measures both concentration and motor speed as subjects are timed when naming successive rows of four coloured squares on each of eight pages.

Mood and emotional status were measured by the Profile of Mood Scales (POMS) an adjectival checklist filled out by the patient (Lorr et al., 1975). A detailed explanation of each of these tests has been described previously (Novelly, 1986; Smith, 1986). Consistency in the administration of the test between sites was assured by training all study assistants in a two-day workshop and by continuous monitoring of results for discrepant values.

CONTROL – EPILEPSY COMPARISONS

The characteristics of both the control group and the patients with epilepsy is shown in Table 2. Education level was ranked from 1 to 8 with 1 representing the highest (PhD) level of education, and 8 representing a grade school level or less. The epilepsy group was slightly older, had fewer females, but had very similar education experience compared with the control group. The patients with epilepsy had a full-scale IQ as measured by the WAIS within an expected normal range. Control subjects were not examined using the WAIS, but because there is such a strong correlation between age, education, and IQ, we felt that these measures were sufficient to match the two groups.

Table 3 shows the correlation found between neuropsychological variables and age, education and IQ among the patients with epilepsy. The negative correlation between education and the behavioural tests reflects the coding of

Table 2.   Control–epilepsy subject characteristics

	Control	Epilepsy
Number	75	618
Mean age	38.6 (13.1)	40.4 (15.3)
Age range	17–72	18–82
Sex (males)	72%	85%
Education (coded)	4.1	4.9
Education range	1–8	1–8
Verbal IQ	NA	100.5 (14.5)
Range		55–142
Performance IQ	NA	99.2 (13.6)
Range		52–134
Full-scale IQ	NA	100.0 (13.5)
Range		52–135

Table 3. Rank-ordered correlations: Age, education, FSIQ (N = 618)

Age		Education		Full-scale IQ	
	R		R		R
Digit symbol	−0.53	Full-scale IQ	−0.47*	Digit span	0.49
Pegboard (total)	0.47	Digit symbol	−0.45	Education	−0.47*
Discriminative reaction time	0.33	Word finding	−0.35	Word finding	0.45
Critical flicker fusion	0.30	Digit span	−0.32	Digit symbol	0.40
		Pegboard (total)	0.31		

* The negative correlation reflects the coding of the education scale from 1 to 9 with the lowest numbers indicating the highest level of education.

the educational scale with the highest numbers indicating the lowest levels of education. Only the highest correlations are shown, and were only computed from tests done during the initial relatively drug-free state. The strong rela-

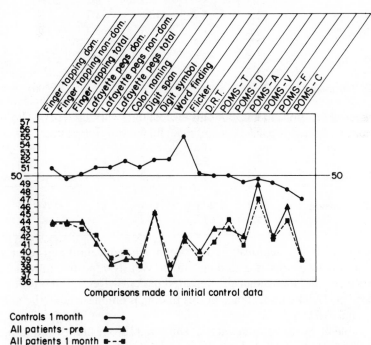

Comparisons made to initial control data

Controls 1 month ●——●
All patients - pre ▲——▲
All patients 1 month ■--■

Fig. 1   In this figure, all the data have been transformed into standardized T score values with a higher score indicating a better performance. The level of performance of the control group at trial I was scaled to 50 and used as a basis for comparison of epilepsy patients at trial I and II, and control subjects at trial II.

Table 4. Control–epilepsy group comparisons for neuropsychological variables: means and standard deviations

Variable	Control subjects (n = 75)		Epilepsy subjects (n = 618)		Control vs. epileptics	
	Trial I	Trial II	Trial I	Trial II	Trial I	Trial II
Tapping total	98.9	99.6	90.0	89.5	<.006	<.0005
	14.6	14.0	16.9	15.6		
Colours	109.8	106.2	137.7	138.8	<.0001	<.0001
	25.4	23.2	43.5	43.5		
Pegboard total	138.4	132.6	177.4	173.9	<.0001	<.0001
	35.5	28.3	56.3	55.9		
Digit span	11.7	12.1	10.6	10.5	>.20	<.003
	2.2	2.3	2.4	2.6		
Digit symbol	59.9	62.3	43.6	44.8	<.0001	<.0001
	12.0	11.8	14.0	14.0		
Word finding	18.5	21.2	14.1	14.2	<.0001	<.0001
	5.7	5.9	5.6	5.8		
CFF	3.5	3.3	8.5	9.1	<.0005	<.001
	4.9	4.2	10.6	11.7		
Reaction time	643.8	651.2	756.1	768.4	<.008	<.002
	139.7	137.2	219.1	216.7		
POMS tension	38.5	39.2	42.8	41.5	<.0002	<.10
	5.7	7.3	8.1	7.6		
POMS depression	37.6	39.0	41.4	41.4	<.0001	<.02
	4.1	5.9	6.5	6.5		
POMS anger	43.3	44.0	44.0	45.2	>.48	>.5
	5.5	7.3	7.5	7.9		
POMS vigour	62.6	61.2	55.8	55.7	<.0001	<.0007
	9.2	9.5	9.8	9.9		
POMS fatigue	44.3	45.3	46.3	47.6	>.18	>.06
	6.7	7.9	8.1	9.0		
POMS confusion	38.2	40.2	44.1	43.3	<.0001	<.019
	5.5	7.2	7.7	7.8		

tionship which was demonstrated between age, education and several of the behavioural measures is a finding not previously reported in patients with epilepsy or other neurologically impaired patients (Reed, 1963; Reitan, 1955; Reitan, 1967). The importance of this finding is emphasized in the analysis of individual AED effects.

In Table 4, the mean values at trial I and trial II (one month of treatment) for the individual neuropsychological tests are shown for both the control subjects, and for patients with epilepsy. Significant differences in performance between the two groups was present for all neuropsychological variables at trial I except for digit span, POMS anger, and POMS fatigue. Fewer differences were found in the POMs test at trial II, but the difference in performance of digit span became significant at trial II. Figure 1 summarizes these same data in a graphic format. In this figure, the data were transformed into standard t values, and the scores of the control group at trial I were scaled to 50 and used as a basis of comparison for controls at trial II, and for patients with epilepsy at both trial I and trial II. Practice effects in the control group can be seen for pegboard, colour naming, digit span, digit symbol and word finding. In contrast, virtually no practice effect was observed in the patient population. Lafayette pegboard and colour naming were particularly effective in discriminating between patients with epilepsy and the control group. On the POMS, epilepsy patients rated themselves higher for tension, depression, confusion and lack of vigour, despite the absence of AED effect.

Perhaps as important, the practice effect noted for the control subjects was not present in the patients with epilepsy when comparing trial I to trial II. The lack of practice effect may be the first indicator of some AED effect.

SPECIFIC EFFECTS OF CBZ, Pb, PRM, AND PHT

The mean number of seizures during the first month and during the first 12 months of monotherapy on CBZ, Pb, PHT, or PRM is shown in Table 5. Although the difference between the mean number of complex partial seizures in the group taking CBZ and the group taking Pb does reach statistical significance, it is doubtful that any difference in seizure frequency among the four patient groups confounds the behavioural data. Seizure type was also uniform among the four groups. Of patients receiving CBZ, 94 had generalized tonic-clonic seizures as opposed to 86 on Pb, 96 on PHT, and 81 on PRM. Sixty-one patients receiving CBZ at entry were classified as having partial seizures, while 69 patients received Pb, 69 PHT, and 66 PRM.

Table 5.   Mean number of seizures

	N	Gen. tonic-clonic	Complex partial
During the first month			
CBZ	103	0.1	3.6
Pb	110	0.3	5.9
PHT	125	0.3	4.0
PRM	96	0.1	2.8
During the first 12 months			
CBZ	63	0.4	3.8
Pb	66	0.6	10.2
PHT	79	0.9	4.6
PRM	50	0.5	6.2

Table 6.   Total behavioural toxicity score for each drug at 1, 3, 6 and 12 months

Month	1	3	6	12
P value	.001	.002	NS	.01
CBZ	15.5	14.9	14.8	16.1
PHT	17.3	20.1	15.9	20.1
Pb	21.3	17.2	15.8	18.5
PRM	17.5	18.5	16.1	18.3

Effects of the four drugs on the behavioural test battery

Examination of the raw scores of all of the subtests for each of the four drug groups at baseline, 3 months, 6 months, and 12 months, revealed no significant trend. Even when rare statistical differences were found, the differences were between the two drugs at each extreme of performance. Only on discrimination reaction time (DRT) at one month was there any apparent meaningful difference with PHT being significantly worse than both Pb and PRM but not significantly different than CBZ. Even this result did not sustain at 6 months and 12 months. Comparing composite scores obtained by grouping the subtests in major areas of neuropsychological function revealed disappointingly few significant differences between the four drugs.

When the total behavioural toxicity battery (BTB) score was calculated, however, a meaningful difference emerged (Table 6). The total BTB score is the result of combining the scores of individual subtests transformed into weighted ordinal units of change based upon published norms.

When no statistical trend for the individual subtests was uncovered, it was elected simply to count the number of best and worst performances on each of the subtests at each rating period. Again, no trend was evident. The same procedure was then used to compare the performance of each of the drugs in patients who were drug naïve at entry into the study. Virtually the same result was obtained as when the entire patient population was studied.

Because of the interrelationships between age, education and IQ found in the initial pre-drug evaluations, the data were then covaried for age and education. Using this method, trends became more apparent. Employing an analysis of variance procedure to assess statistical significance, the group of patients on CBZ scored better than at least two other AED groups on pegboard at 3 months, finger tap and digit span at 6 months, and digit span at 12 months with a confidence level of >0.005. The groups taking Pb or PRM scored worse on pegboard at 3 months, digit span at 12 months, and digit symbol at both 6 and 12 months. These differences were apparent whether examining raw scores, change scores, or the simplified approach of simply counting the number of best and worst performances. This finding emphasizes the need to consider the effects of age and education when evaluating be-

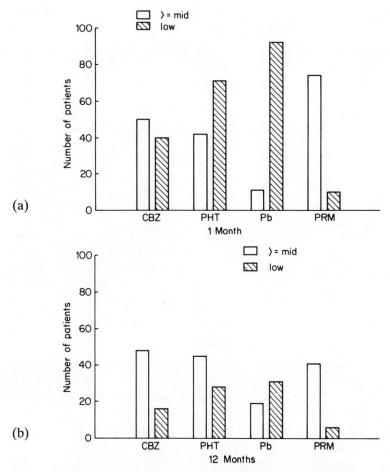

Fig. 2   The total number of patients in the sub or low therapeutic range compared with the total number of patients in the mid–high excess range for each drug at 1 month (a) and at 12 months (b).

havioural measures, and points out the errors that can be generated unless age, education and general intellectual ability are carefully controlled. When age and education were *not* covaried, even change scores failed to reveal any consistent pattern, although the change scores for digit symbol seemed most sensitive in separating the barbiturates from PHT and CBZ.

We then examined the relationship of serum blood level within the individual subtest scores by drug. No differences for any drug even on the total BTB score reached statistical significance. That is, no statistically significant difference in scores for any drug group could be detected when patients in the low and sub-therapeutic ranges were compared with patients in the mid to high and excess ranges. However, when the *number* of patients achieving serum drug levels in the low and subrange of accepted therapeutic values (CBZ < 6 micrograms/cc; Pb <25 micrograms/cc; PHT < 14 micrograms/cc; and PRM <6 micrograms/cc) was compared with the number of patients achieving serum levels equal to or greater than mid therapeutic range (CBZ > = 7; Pb > = 26; PHT > 15; and PRM > = 7 micrograms/cc) at each rating period, dramatic differences were apparent. Figure 2 compares the mean antiepileptic blood level for each group at one and 12 months. More patients on both PRM and CBZ had levels in the 'mid' and 'high' therapeutic ranges at both rating periods than did either PHT or Pb. The difference is particularly striking when comparing Pb and PRM. Given the huge discrepancy in the number of patients between groups, it is little wonder that no statistical significance could be determined with regard to difference in performance based on blood levels. The discrepancy in numbers, however, may in itself be highly meaningful. The fact that there were so many patients in the mid, high, excess range who were taking either PRM or CBZ, suggests that it was relatively easy to increase the dosages of these two drugs without inducing intolerable toxicity. Conversely, the large number of patients in the Pb group in the sub to low range suggests that it was difficult to increase the dose of Pb into the mid-high range. Similar, but less striking numbers are present in the group taking PHT (Figure 2).

SUMMARY

The ability to examine a large number of patients with well-documented and classified seizures who were relatively drug-free is a unique feature of this study. The strict exclusion criteria used at entry and the fact that the patients with epilepsy in this study were otherwise healthy, and their seizures were not intractable, adds significance to the behavioural profile obtained. In contrast to this study, previous studies have reported that patients with epilepsy have lower levels of general intellectual performance than the general population (Lennox, 1942; Matthews and Kløve, 1967; Kløve and Matthews, 1969; Dodrill and Troupin, 1974; Reynolds, 1983). It has been difficult to interpret these reports because of the confounding effects of AEDs and the inclusion of chronic uncontrolled epilepsy patients. In this study, the mean IQ of the patients was 100.0 ± 13.5, well within the range expected in the general population. None the less, these patients demonstrated significant differences in performances on subtests of the BTB used in this study when compared with a group of controls carefully matched for age, sex and education.

Despite the large number of patients and the careful study design which eliminated many of the confounding variables inherent in previous studies, when the raw data were examined, no dramatic differences in the performance of patients taking CBZ, Pb, PRM or PHT were found. As expected, the barbiturates fared somewhat less well overall than did CBZ or PHT, but even this difference rarely reached statistical significance. When the results of all of the subtests were combined in the total BTB score, significant differences between the four drugs emerged. CBZ consistently had less effect on cognitive function as measured by this test battery than Pb, PHT, or PRM at all rating periods. This finding confirms the results of other studies (Trimble, Chapter 10) which have indicated that CBZ has fewer cognitive effects than PHT or the barbiturates. Perhaps more importantly, this study emphasizes the need to control for age, education and IQ when assessing individual neuropsychological test results.

Even though the total toxicity battery did reveal some differences in the cognitive effects of these four drugs, the most striking finding is that there were so few meaningful differences in the individual subtests. It is likely that when patients are managed by experienced 'epileptologists', adverse effects of AEDs are minized. This, combined with a study design which encouraged physicians to lower the dose when 'unacceptable' toxicity intervened resulted in a very different subject population (i.e. patients who were well managed from the onset) than in previous reports and provides an explanation for the struggle, evident in this paper, to extract statistically meaningful differences between the four AEDs.

ACKNOWLEDGEMENTS

The author acknowledges the contributions of: R.H. Mattson, J. Cramer, P.D. Williamson, R. Novelly (West Haven, CT); R.B. Craft (Augusta, GA); T.R. Browne (Boston, MA); R. Homan (Dallas, TX); J.O. McNamara (Durham, NC); D. Treiman, A. Delgado-Escueta (Los Angeles, CA); M.F. Lubozynski, A. Mayersdorf (Minneapolis, MN); C.B. McCutchen (San Diego, CA); W.E. Crill (Seattle, WA); and J.B. Collins (Perry Point, MD).

REFERENCES

CRAMER, J.A., SMITH, D.B., MATTSON, R.H., DELGADO ESCUETA, A.V. and COLLINS, J.F. (1983) A method of quantification for the evaluation of antiepileptic drug therapy. *Neurology*, **33(1)**, 26–37.

DELGADO ESCUETA, A.V., MATTSON, R.H., SMITH, D.B., CRAMER, J.A. and COLLINS, J.F. (1983) Principles in designing clinical trials for antiepileptic drugs. *Neurology*, **33(1)**, 8–13.

DODRILL, C.B. (1981) Neuropsychology of epilepsy. In *Handbook of Clinical Neuropsychology* (eds S.B. FILSKOV and T.J. BOLL), pp. 366–395, John Wiley, New York.

DODRILL, C.B. and TROUPIN, A.S. (1974) Effects of repeated administration of a comprehensive neuropsychological battery among chronic epileptics. *J. Nerv. Ment. Dis.*, **161**, 185–190.

KLØVE, H. and MATTHEWS, C.G.L. (1969) Neuropsychological evaluation of the epileptic patient. *Wis. Med. J.*, 68, 296–301.

LENNOX, W.G. (1942) Brain injury, drugs and environment as causes of mental decay in epilepsy. *Am. J. Psychiatry*, **99**, 174–180.

LEWIS, R.F. and RENNICK, P.M. (1979) *Manual for the Repeatable Cognitive-Perceptual-Motor Battery*, Axon, Grosse Point, Michigan.

LORR, J., McNAIR, D.M. and DROPPLEMAN, L.F. (1971) *Manual: Profile of Mood States*, Educational and Industrial Testing Service, San Diego, California.

MATTHEWS, C.G. and KLØVE, H. (1967) Differential psychological performances in major motor, psychomotor and mixed seizure classification of known and unknown etiology. *Epilepsia*, **8**, 117–128.

MATTSON, R.H. (1983) The design of clinical studies to assess the efficacy and toxicity of antiepileptic drugs. *Neurology*, **33**, 1–37.

MATTSON, R.H., CRAMER, J.A., COLLINS, J.F. and SMITH, D.B. (1985) VA Cooperative Study 118 Group. Comparison of carbamazepine, phenobarbital, phenytoin, and primidone in partial and secondary generalized tonic-clonic seizures. *N. Engl. J. Med.*, **313**, 145–151.

NOVELLY, R.A., SCHUMARTZ, M.M., MATTSON, R.H. and CRAMER, J.A. (1986) Behavioral toxicity associated with antiepileptic drugs: Concepts and methods of assessment. *Epilepsia, 27*, 331–340.

REED, H.B.C., Jr and REITAN, R.M. (1963) Changes in psychological test performance associated with the normal aging process. *J. Gerontol.*, **18**, 271–274.

REITAN, R.M. (1955) The distribution according to age of a psychologic measure dependent upon organic brain functions. *J. Gerontol.*, **10**, 338–340.

REITAN, R.M. (1967) Psychological changes associated with aging and with cerebral damage. *Mayo Clin. Proc.*, **42**, 653–673.

REITAN, R.M. and DAVIDSON, L.A. (1974) *Clinical Neuropsychology: Current Status and Applications*. Hemisphere, New York.

REYNOLDS, E.H. (1983) Mental effects of antiepileptic medication. *Epilepsia*, **24**, S85–S95.

SMITH, D.B., CRAFT, B.R., COLLINS, J., MATTSON, R.H., CRAMER, J.A. and the VA Cooperative Study Group 118 (1986) Behavioral characteristics of epilepsy patients compared with normal controls. *Epilepsia*, **27**, 760–768.

Discussion

Section II

Dr D.B. Smith: Dr Binnie, were there any subjects who had discharges, who didn't have any detectable change in their cognitive function during discharges, and if so, did they differ in any other respect from the subjects who did have such disturbances?

Dr C.D. Binnie: Yes, we were able to demonstrate TCI in 50% of the people we tested. Other authors have come up with the roughly the same figure. However, in spite of our method of selection, screening out all the people who had overt clinical manifestations on the CCTV or who showed the classical kind of EEG abnormality which is supposed to produce TCI. We still got 50% of our patients showing TCI. Whether different tasks would show effects in the others, we cannot tell, but the very fact that the effects are task-specific to some extent, particularly in relation to the focal discharges, suggests that one does need to try other tasks. We did define 'epileptiform activity' for this purpose rather widely, and we found that patients who had episodic delta activity did not show TCI.

Dr P.B.C. Fenwick: Dr Smith, what were the phenobarbitone levels in the primidone group? Were they very much lower than the phenobarbitone levels in the phenobarbitone group?

Dr D.B. Smith: They were significantly lower.

Dr M. Harper (Cardiff): Dr Reynolds in his presentation was sceptical of the concept of sustained behavioural disturbances in the absence of definite fits as being anything to do with epilepsy. However, if you combine the evidence of cognitive impairment in subclinical states with the evidence from depth electrode studies are we still right to maintain that only brief and episodic disturbances of behaviour can be regarded as epilepsy?

Dr P.B.C. Fenwick: That is a very exciting question and it's right at the basis of where our thinking of epileptic discharges is at the present time. It seems to me that the old idea that there were such things as epileptic equivalents has come right back into fashion. The fact that you can observe seizure discharges occurring in the depth and only minimal changes in scalp recordings, producing very profound alterations of behaviour opens up this whole area. It is no longer thought to be an occasional occurrence. There are two reasons for this: you can get behavioural changes at the onset of seizures which occur in association with depth discharges before the seizure spreads. Secondly, episodes of

79

behavioural change are seen in actual seizures which are confined to the depth. All the temporal lobe research groups using depth electrodes have reported this, and seizures confined to the amygdala or hippocampus are common. Also, you can get frontal lobe seizures confined electrically to the frontal lobes, without changes on the scalp. So the whole question now of discharges within the depth producing paroxysmal disorders of behaviour is open.

Dr C.D. Binnie: The available evidence on depth recording in people showing episodic disorder of behaviour other than epileptic seizures is very limited. For obvious ethical reasons, it is difficult to obtain. It is true that one can have electrical discharges in the depth which are not seen on the surface. But these are not usually manifest by behavioural changes. They are typically associated with simple partial experiences. The patient may be experiencing déjà vu, or some other sensation, and not usually behaving abnormally.

Dr P.B.C. Fenwick: That is absolutely right. But it's the principle that you can't get behavioural changes with discharges in the depth which is important.

Dr D.B. Smith: Dr Binnie, you showed there that there was a great deal of impairment prior to the electrical discharge that you recorded on the surface. I wonder if that might be a manifestation of the beginning of the discharge in the depth that is responsible for that impairment?

Dr C.D. Binnie: This seems the likeliest explanation. This has been looked at in many studies of TCI. Most of them haven't found anything prior to the onset of discharge. One study claimed an improvement. We only found impairment in the children doing the reading task. One might say, these were children having partial epilepsy where one has good evidence that the discharge can be localized to deep structures, but we saw that equally with partial and generalized seizures.

Dr J. Brown (Edinburgh): Dr Fenwick, do you think there is such a thing as a primary generalized seizure at all?

Dr P.B.C. Fenwick: Are we right in thinking that there is such a condition as primary generalized epilepsy? The answer is, probably not; except with a spontaneous seizure related only to genetic causes, but how common are they? Probably relatively uncommon. My reason for saying that is that every new diagnostic method that has come along has reduced the number of people with epilepsy where cerebral change of some sort is not found. With depth electrodes for example, where there are petit mal absences and seizures of a primary generalized type, then we see that there are areas of the brain which lead to discharges, and produce exactly those features of the seizure that we thought to be genetic before. I suspect that this process of contraction will continue, and there will be an ever smaller group of patients who have true genetic seizures.

Dr D.B. Smith: There are many studies in which the brain is well covered with depth and surface electrodes recording simultaneously up to 180 channels, and in some instances you see a generalized onset. It is impossible, even with computer techniques to detect a sequencing. I find it almost impossible to conceptualize how all areas of the brain could start to discharge simultaneously, there must be a focus that somehow we are missing. Perhaps because we do not impale the thalamus, for ethical reasons.

Dr C.D. Binnie: Could I also respond, not so much in aetiological or pathological terms, as in neurophysiological terms. Since the Montreal School introduced their model of the generalized cortical epilepsies we have been asked to believe that primary generalized epilepsy involves diffuse cortical hyperexcitability and that the hyperexcitable cortex responds abnormally to normal physiological inputs. Now it is a very small step to suggest that the cortical hyperexcitability does not have to be uniform, and if it isn't uniform, it will start in one place before it starts somewhere else. Evidence of non-uniformity of cortical hyperexcitability is difficult to find, I can offer only one example, and that is in photosensitive patients, many of whom have primary generalized epilepsy; a lot are pattern sensitive. If you present patterns to one half-visual field you elicit the discharges in the contra-lateral visual temporal region. You can demonstrate, in many of these patients with primary generalized epilepsy, that the threshold for stimulation by pattern is lower in one hemisphere than the other. On the Montreal model, this suggests to me that the cortical hyperexcitability which they postulate does not have to be uniform, and probably usually isn't. In which case, all generalized seizures with start focally somewhere.

Dr C. Verity (Cambridge): I'm asked by paediatricians to give an opinion on children who have unusual behaviours which may or may not be epilepsy. One of the questions which they ask is to what extent is prolonged EEG monitoring going to help. In view of what you have been saying, are we just going to be misleading ourselves if we are only using surface electrodes?

Dr C.D. Binnie: It all depends on the nature of the seizure. If the patient has a simple partial seizure, particularly a simple partial seizure with only psychic or sensory symptoms and the EEG does not change, this is not a cause for concern. If however he shows other kinds of symptomatology which do normally produce scalp EEG changes, and the EEG does not change, you can say that this is not an epileptic seizure. If he seems to have an absence and the EEG does not change, in my opinion that was not an epileptic seizure. You do need good documentation of the behaviour. There is a lot to be said for videotelemetry rather than sending the patient off into the wild with a tape recorder and not knowing what really has happened.

Professor N. O'Donohoe (Dublin): In benign partial epilepsy, which is probably one of the commonest forms of epilepsy in adolescents, areas of localized cortical hyperexcitability seem to come in a mysterious way and disappear again after years, often with very few seizures occurring. Nobody has yet succeeded in demonstrating any structural abnormality; there appears to be abnormality of 'function', if you like. As a paediatric neurologist, I would certainly hang on grimly to the concept of primary epilepsy, which has yet to be shown as false.

Dr C.D. Binnie: We never saw benign childhood epilepsy when I was at a special centre in Holland. When I got back in England, one of the first things that I wanted to do was to see whether we could demontrate TCI during these spikes, and you can.

Dr M.R. Trimble: What name would Dr Fenwick give to those events in which a patient has symptoms of abnormal behaviour and clearly discharging abnormalities within deep structures of the brain?

Dr P.B.C. Fenwick: The answer depends on the question of when is a neural discharge abnormal and of sufficient length to be called epilepsy? The discharges which I was talking about, the ones that Heath characterized, were seizure discharges, prolonged bursts of abnormal activity within the depths and one would call those 'seizures'. They were not always limited to the depths, at other times they would spread out of the depths and produce characteristic seizure patterns in the scalp EEG. I will be happy to stick with 'seizure discharges' in the limbic system for the time being.

Dr E.H. Reynolds: It is partly a semantic issue, but it has enormous practical implications. It does not surprise me if behavioural disturbances or other clinical phenomena such as involuntary movement disorders have as their basis abnormal neuronal discharges. However, I do not think it right to call all abnormal electrical discharges 'epilepsy'. The reason some people call these 'epilepsy' or 'seizure discharges' is because Jackson said epilepsy is 'excessive neuronal discharge'. But Jackson backed off his neurophysiological definition and I suggest that we too should restrict the term epilepsy to a clinical concept. Otherwise, like Jackson and others, we are in danger of seeing epilepsy everywhere, or in danger of using confusing terms such as epileptoid, larval epilepsy, etc. Let us stick to neutral terms, such as 'discharges'. We still have to learn the relationship between these electrical discharges and the clinical entities that we are interested in.

Dr J. Green (Manchester): Dr Binnie, there was a time when we used to talk about three cycle per second spike wave as the common abnormality in simple epilepsies, but nowadays we talk about atypical spike-wave or atypical spike and poly-spike. Are these two groups different, from a neurophysiological point of view?

Dr C.D. Binnie: There seems, unfortunately, to be a continuum, from the patients who have typical absences, who have typical spike-wave and a family history of epilepsy, through to patients who are very atypical who have episodes of alteration of consciousness which could be either absences or complex partial seizures, which do not respond to the usual drugs for absence seizures or partial seizures, and their EEG shows patterns between the two. Within, at least, the official classification you have the many variants. The more you depart from the classical absence of just staring and eye-lid fluttering and have changes in muscle tone and so on, the more likely you are to see the more complex wave forms.

Dr H.J. Sagar (Sheffield): Dr Smith, if one accepts that there is an association between the toxic and the cognitive effects of a drug then it is not surprising that one does not see much difference between the drugs from the way that your study was designed. In all cases you backed off from a point defined by toxicity. This point need not be equivalent in terms of drug levels or effect on seizure control. Do you have any information on the differences on the cognitive tests under conditions of equivalent effect on seizure control?

Dr D.B. Smith: We backed off on the basis of clinical toxicity and were hoping that the neuro-psychological tests might be a bit more sophisticated than our clinical judgement or the patient's self-reporting of intolerable toxicity. We tried to look at a more homogeneous grouping by eliminating all of those patients within the toxic range, but we still did not see any great differences between the drugs; we took those patients within the defined mid-therapeutic range. In terms of seizure control, there were differences between the drugs that were significant for partial complex seizures. When measuring seizure control in terms of absolute control, absence of seizures for one year on monotherapy with a single anti-epileptic drug, carbamazepine, was significantly better in controlling complex partial seizures than any of the other three drugs. There was no difference however, in the control of generalized tonic-clonic seizures after one year on mono-therapy, between the four drugs.

Dr H.J. Sagar: But are you able to say whether there is any difference in the cognitive performance in those groups that are equated for seizure control across the drugs?

Dr D.B. Smith: I think that the groups were quite comparable in terms of seizure control. So I do not think that that is a meaningful variable.

Ms J. Ossetin: Dr Smith, if someone had seizure control, why did you not reduce the dose?

Dr D.B. Smith: We were hoping to be able to determine whether or not the accepted therapeutic ranges were in fact accurate. I think what we did show was that the therapeutic ranges for both primidone and carbamazepine, as given in 1978 when the study began, were considerably lower than what is accurate. It is necesary in many patients to push up doses and one can do so without significant toxicity to a serum level in the low teens (micrograms/ml) for carbamazepine and for primidone.

Ms J. Ossetin: But were you pushing up only if seizure control was not achieved?

Dr D.B. Smith: No. Even if seizure control was achieved, it was our purpose to push up doses but that did not always occur. There were ten centres, and not every investigator did that well, but that was the intent of the study. The blood levels do show that this was to a large extent achieved. One of the objectives of the study was to assess relative toxicity of the various drugs, and to try to assess the therapeutic ranges of those drugs. The problem is, of course, it is going to self select, and to some extent that is shown by the result with phenobarbitone. That levelled out to a much lower level, presumably because of the greater toxicity. The textbooks quote a 20–40 micrograms per ml range, but it is the rare patient who can tolerate phenobarbitone much above the mid-twenties.

Section III

7

Educational needs and epilepsy in childhood

EUAN M. ROSS and PAT TOOKEY
Charing Cross Hospital and Institute of Child Health, London

INTRODUCTION

Making confident general statements about the special needs of this diverse group of children with different seizure types and severity of epilepsy is precarious. Those with other handicaps as well as epilepsy tend to do badly whatever outcome measures are used; in contrast, those educated in the normal system do reasonably well. This raises questions – does education in a mainstream as opposed to a special school influence eventual ability? Are the problems that children with epilepsy attract intrinsically due to seizures and attempts to control them with drugs, or are they a reflection of the underlying instability of the brain which leads to seizure disorder? Large whole community-based studies can shed some light on these issues.

The education of children with epilepsy has to be seen in the context of current debates about schooling: these centre on the curriculum, the integration or otherwise of the handicapped into mainstream schools and the role of parental choice and their influence in education. Informed decision-making requires properly conducted research. Although a considerable amount of work has been done on the subject of epilepsy and education, many of its results are scattered in research reports, abstracts of meetings and monographs and relatively little in readily available medical literature.

Sources of data

The descriptions of childhood epilepsy in standard medical textbooks mainly stem from teaching hospital experience. They tend not to draw their patients from a true cross-section of the population and may over represent those with highly complex or atypical disorders. High social class parents tend to seek out the more famous hospitals; this was well demonstrated by the child population with epilepsy attending the Maida Vale Hospital, London described by Bagley (1971).

In England and Wales about 400 children with epilepsy (perhaps 0.5–1% of those affected) are educated in special residential schools for epilepsy. Morgan and Kurtz (1986) discussed them in detail and they are not discussed further in this chapter.

Understanding of epilepsy among other handicapping conditions in whole communities was greatly expanded through community-based studies. These included the postwar Newcastle 1000 family study (Miller et al., 1974), the Isle of Wight study of all schoolchildren on that island by Rutter et al. (1972), and the specific studies of epilepsy in children attending normal schools in Bedfordshire by Holdsworth and Whitmore (1974) and in London by Kangesu et al. (1984). Other important large-scale epilepsy studies have been undertaken in Iceland (Gudmundsson, 1966); Finland (Sillaanpaa, 1973) and the United States (Ellenberg et al., 1986). An intensive epidemiological review was made by Zielinsky (1982).

The most complete British national overview of epilepsy in unselected schoolchildren comes from the National Child Development Study (NCDS) in which the ante and perinatal histories of virtually all 17,733 children born in the week 3–9 March 1958 in England, Scotland and Wales were documented. The techniques used and a summary of the findings were published by Ross et al. (1980); Ross and Peckham (1983); and Kurtz, Tookey and Ross (1987). The survivors were traced to their schools at ages 7, 11 and 16 where they were medically examined, school performance assessed and parents visited by health visitors who recorded their socio-medical histories. At 23 the cohort was again traced to their homes and socio-medical interviews undertaken. Those with any evidence of epilepsy either first reported then, or in the earlier phases of the study were found to have had fits after age 16 are currently being interviewed at home and – subject to their consent – their doctors have been asked to give up-to-date medical information.

Further British information about child development and epilepsy from unselected cohort samples comes from the two other national studies based on all children born in England, Scotland and Wales in single weeks in the spring of 1946 (Cooper, 1965, 1970; Verity and Ross, 1985); further data about the ability of school children with epilepsy are awaited from the latter study.

Epilepsies in school-aged children

The NCDS (Ross et al., 1980) showed that:

• The overall prevalence of epilepsy (at least two nonfebrile seizures after the first week of life) in school-aged children in the UK is of the order of 4–5 children per 1000.

- A further 2 per 1000 children have been labelled as having epilepsy by at least one doctor but there is reasonable doubt concerning the reliability of the diagnosis.
- About half the children with epilepsy have not had a fit in the past two years. Their epilepsy is 'quiescent' as distinct from the further 2–3 per 1000 with fits in the past two years classified as 'active epilepsy'.

Possible causes

Taking all types of epilepsy and severity together, a cause could be found for about 25% of cases in the NCDS, about half of which might have been prevented with better care or better luck. Subsequent improvements in neonatal and paediatric care have lowered these figures. Ross and Bommen (1983) in a more recent hospital-based series found no potentially preventable cause for epilepsy among children who were born in the UK, though several were due to preventable illness in developing countries.

The following list based on findings from the 1958 and 1970 British National Studies suggests an approximate breakdown of the clinical seizure patterns that might be found in a British schoolchild population:

	%
Grand mal	50
Benign focal rolandic	15
Psychomotor or temporal lobe	10
Pattern or flicker-induced	10
Classical petit mal	2
Myoclonic seizures	5
Other types	8

Since misconceptions are commonly made about even the more common epilepsy syndromes, it is important that doctors appreciate the common pitfalls:

Petit mal epilepsy is rare and too often overdiagnosed. The term should be reserved for those with classic absence attacks without further features. Too many doctors, let alone lay people, incorrectly refer to any short fit as petit mal. Parents deserve truthful information. They will read about epilepsy and may come away with confused messages. Most short seizures are grand mal in type but modified with treatment.

Temporal lobe seizures are typically manifest by a short outburst of abnormal uncoordinated behaviour. Clinically typical cases can be found despite lack of characteristic EEG changes. Affected children usually function in the mentally normal range but may develop bizarre defence mechanisms that try the patience of their parents, teachers and friends; close cooperation between paediatrician and child psychiatrist is needed.

Benign congenital focal Rolandic seizures. These benign fits in sleeping children often greatly alarm parents who may need a great deal of counselling. Their course is usually self-limiting and rarely persists after childhood. The condition is often unrecognized by doctors; overtreatment with anticonvulsants must be avoided.

Pattern or flicker associated seizures. Only a small minority of children with epilepsy have fits provoked by flicker. Many children spend hours in front of television screens and it should not be assumed that all fits in these circumstances are due to photosensitivity (Wilkins, 1987). A large London Further Education College recently banned all pupils with epilepsy from undertaking computer studies. There is no evidence however that special computer monitor screens (as distinct from domestic televisions hooked to a computer) are a practical cause of flicker associated seizures (Binnie et al., 1985). These facts need to be known within schools and colleges.

It is becoming increasingly apparent that the unifying term 'epilepsy' is becoming less useful as more and more discrete seizure disorders are being recognized. It is now essential to attempt to describe the disorder both in terms of aetiology and clinical features. They are well described in the recent textbook by Aicardi (1986) and in a symposium report edited by Roger et al. (1985). Both include accounts of a large number of epileptic syndromes, many of which have only been described in recent years. Typical conditions associated with epilepsy include Rett, Fragile X, and Landau-Kleffner syndromes, *inter alia.* 'New' causes of seizure disorder are being recognized, the most important being AIDS which causes a wide variety of neurodegenerative signs. Many seizure patterns do not follow textbook descriptions. There are not enough doctors available to the school health service who have the experience and up-to-date knowledge to recognize the rarer or more recently recognized syndromes. Geneticists should be encouraged to visit special schools in order to help diagnose children with unexplained syndromes. Knowing the name of the child's syndrome helps parents to cease their quest for a cause and concentrate on treatment.

Social factors

The NCDS (and other studies) show that as a group one-parent families were over-represented, but of those in complete families the social class distribution was similar among controls. In a study of secondary schoolchildren in Bristol,

Ross (1975) found that divorce and death of one parent, particularly fathers, was more common than expected, reflecting the burden thrown by a handicapped child onto the family which may break it. The National Childhood Encephalopathy Study (Miller et al., 1985) found that among children with a serious neurological disorder in their first three years there is an 11-fold increase in risk of at least one parent having a neurological or psychiatric disorder.

Educational performance and school placement

The NCDS found that one-third of children with substantiated epilepsy were receiving special education, the majority were in special schools with only a few getting special help in normal schools. Subsequently the concept of 'special needs' was introduced following the implementation of the 1981 Education Act. It is now mandatory that any child who requires extra educational provision has a statement of special educational need drawn up. All professionally concerned and the parents are asked to write about the child's needs from their standpoint. These 'statements' are read by the parent and submitted to the educational authorities who are obliged to offer appropriate educational provision. This is open to appeal by the parents. There are considerable advantages to the child and family as long as the scheme is correctly implemented. This process is centred on needs not diagnosis so it does not lend itself to the collection of descriptive data about epilepsy or other handicapping disorder.

Epilepsy on its own is not a common reason for special education. Of the 21 in the NCDS at special school with epilepsy at age 11, the commonest associated problem was mental handicap (9), though a wide variety of problems was found including behaviour problems (3), cerebral palsy (2) and deafness (1). Three were in special education principally on account of epilepsy.

The NCDS showed that children with epilepsy who attended special schools generally made dismal intellectual achievements, reflecting the severity of mental handicap. It was not possible to determine the influence of epilepsy on the achievements of this group. It is probable that their performance would have been retarded even if there had never been any seizures. Most were unable to get employment on leaving school though there were occasional encouragements including a champion shot put in international games for the handicapped. Whilst there is a need for properly controlled studies which would assess rates of progress among children with epilepsy attending mainstream or special schools, epilepsy *per se* may be one of the least important problems to the family of a severely handicapped child.

The child with epilepsy at normal school

Two-thirds of affected children in the NCDS were educated in the normal school system. As a group at age 11 their maths, reading and general ability scores were slightly lower but within one SD of the mean for the study. Behavioural characteristics show a group who are bullied rather than bullying, meek and showing less aggression than noted by teachers for the study as a whole. The mean Bristol Social Adjustment Guide Score at age seven was however higher (more unsettled) both in those children who had already had two or more fits *and* in those who were going to present with epilepsy in the period when they were aged between 7 to 11 years, than in those who never had fits. This finding suggests that some brain disturbance, enough to alter social adjustment, may be present before fits present (see Table 1).

Table 1. Bristol social adjustment score aged 7 (as %)

	Settled (0–9)	Unsettled (10+)
First fit pre-7 years n = 38	38	62
First fit after 7 years n = 14	43	57
Remainder n = 14 905	64	36

Investigation

Diagnosis starts with the history including an eye-witness account of the seizures followed by a detailed examination. This requires no special facilities apart from a doctor prepared to examine the child adequately. The child must be completely undressed so that skin signs such as the café au lait patches of tuberous sclerosis can be found; optic fundi, blood pressure and growth chart must be studied. The child must be observed for long enough in an attempt to witness seizures.

The role of special investigations is becoming clearer but many fail to appreciate that the diagnosis of epilepsy is clinical and is not made by EEG or CT scan which are but adjuncts to the skill of the clinician. In practice most children in the UK with suspected seizures now get an electroencephalogram (EEG); a simultaneous video may capture otherwise occult seizures. An average 20-minute recording may miss intermittent episodes of abnormal rhythm and if more information is required a 24-hour portable recording may be needed. This has the benefit of including normal sleep. The quality of recording and interpretation varies widely. The EEG is a useful diagnostic adjunct but diagnosis rests on informed clinical opinion.

Computer assisted tomography (CT scan) greatly facilitates the diagnosis of tuberous sclerosis, enlarged ventricles and tumours though the latter are rare causes of epilepsy in childhood and there is little need for scanning in the absence of clinical suspicion of these disorders such as focal neurological or skin signs or abnormal head growth (Green, 1987). Newer techniques including cerebral function mapping and nuclear magnetic resonance are not yet widely available but are unlikely to be needed in the majority of children with epilepsy.

Management

Drugs are but one element of management. The doctor who starts them has a duty to see they are stopped when they have served their purpose. Their role in cognitive function is discussed by Cull (Chapter 8) and by Corbett et al. (1985). The length of treatment after the last fit will remain more a matter of judgement than science until studies of randomized treatment currently underway are completed. Many series show that only about 50% of children take or are given anticonvulsant drugs as prescribed. There is no point in pressing drugs on reluctant parents or children if they are likely to take them erratically. There is little place for a trial of medication.

Monotherapy is the best policy. Used in combination anticonvulsants tend to antagonize each other and other drugs. Often the use of multiple anticonvulsants is a counsel of despair and the child will be found to make better intellectual progress on a single anticonvulsant. It is rare that increasing dosage to the upper theoretical limit is helpful. Sometimes one drug is vastly better than another yet there are no hard-and-fast rules that foretell which, if any, will be the most effective in a particular child. 'Well-being' rather than cessation of seizures is the goal of treatment.

Phenobarbitone is not a good drug for children because it makes so many irritable and some unmanageable. Phenytoin has the disadvantage of causing gum hypertrophy, abnormal facial growth, excess body hair and continuing anxieties about folate metabolism. Ethosuximide is only known to be effective in classical petit mal though has never been fully investigated for other types of epilepsy.

Currently four drugs are widely used to treat epilepsy in children:

Primidone, a relatively 'old' drug, a variant of phenobarbitone which appears to cause less irritability.
Sodium valproate, as a general purpose anticonvulsant, particularly effective in petit mal and grand mal seizures.
Carbamazepine was initially promoted as a treatment for temporal lobe epilepsy though is now regarded as valuable in most types of childhood epilepsy, apart from classic petit mal.
Clonazepam is a long-acting benzodiazepine; the fact that it has tended to be reserved for more obscure and difficult forms of seizure disorder has limited

practical experience in its use as a first-line anticonvulsant in straightforward cases.

The NCDS and the 1970 birth cohort follow-up in the Child Health and Development Study (CHES) confirm earlier findings that many schoolchildren with epilepsy in the United Kingdom have unfilled special needs. Although national cohort studies have not been undertaken recently, McInlay (1987) reviewed studies which show that this still applies. The key to filling these needs lies in parents, doctors, teachers, nurses, therapists and many other groups professionally involved and working together. This needs good coordination which is greatly helped by an effective District Handicap Team or its equivalent which can bring these many individuals together; the educational and practical liaison work of a specialist nurse for the handicapped can transform care. Having a child with epilepsy places great strains on parents. They can be greatly helped if they are, or can be motivated to learn as much as possible about their own child's problems and learn how to tackle them effectively.

The question of special epilepsy clinics has been raised in the reports of government committees at 15-year intervals since the war, the latest being published in 1986 by HMSO. Despite recommendations (which have never been supported by earmarked finance) only a handful of such clinics have been set up and few children are within easy access of one.

Communication with schools

Some parents wish to keep their child's epilepsy a secret. This poses a potential danger to the child and needless problems for school staff if they have not been told and prepared for seizures to occur. Doctors must encourage the parents to share the problem with the school. One method is for the doctor to phone the school with the permission and in the presence of the parents. This demonstrates to the parents that doctor and school must share information. The key is to let parents hear the conversation and if possible arrange a three-way conversation. It is also useful if the doctor dictates a letter to the school in the presence and with the help of the parents; it is most unusual for parents to decline to let information be shared in this way. Visiting the school and sharing information directly with the teachers, school nurse and parents is the best way to communicate. There is a case for parent-held files that would combine their own with medical and educational records.

Although special education can be extended to age 19, leaving school often coincides with handover of specialist medical care from paediatricians to adult-centred services and much family support is lost simultaneously. The whole burden of care for the young person with handicapping epilepsy may now be thrown back on to the parents. Of 13 in the NCDS with a history of epilepsy and in special education at age 11, 10 had at least one fit after age 23. In contrast of 33 in normal education at age 11, only eight had fits after age 23. For those who are still having fits, job finding is difficult and only those who received a good enough education will be in a favourable position. For those with continuing epilepsy but few learnt skills, employment prospects are bleak.

CONCLUSION

Improving medical services

One of the virtues of the 1974 NHS reorganization and the partial implementation of some of the Court report proposals (DHSS, 1976) has been the creation of consultant paediatricians to the community child health service – about one third of districts now have at least one in post. It is vital that these paediatricians have had on appointment a substantial element of paediatric neurology and child psychiatry in their training in order to bring a wide experience in the diagnosis and treatment of handicap to the school health service. Generally the medical supervision of handicapped children should be done at school though copies of correspondence and clinical records must be kept in the hospital notes and available if the child has to be admitted. There are too few child neurologists in the UK to provide an ongoing service for children with epilepsy; rightly their efforts have to be put into the diagnosis and treatment of the rarer neurological problems that are best managed in hospital where they can contribute to the management of the relatively few children with unstable epilepsies.

Optimal care is most likely when parents, teachers and older children have a clear understanding about the nature of the child's particular form of epilepsy, the rationale of treatment and prognosis. This can only be imparted by doctors. The majority of children who are not otherwise handicapped 'grow out' of their epilepsy and clinicians can often afford to be cautiously optimistic, whilst appreciating that in a growing child symptoms can readily change and periodic re-examination and reassessment are needed whilst the seizure tendency is active.

ACKNOWLEDGEMENTS

The follow-up of children with epilepsy in the National Child Development Study is being carried out at the Institute of Child Health, London with Prof. C. Peckham and Dr Z. Kurtz in cooperation with the National Children's Bureau, London. We are also grateful to Dr S. Jazeel, Principal Physician in Child Health, Riverside Health District, London for helpful advice over school health issues.

REFERENCES

AICARDI, J. (1986) *Epilepsy in Children*. Raven Press, New York.
BAGLEY, C.R. (1971) *Social Psychology of the Child with Epilepsy*. Routledge & Kegan Paul, London.

BINNIE, C.D., TRENITE, D.G.A. K.-N., KORTE, R. de. and WILKINS, A. (1985) Visual display units and risk of seizures. *Lancet*, **i**, 991.

COOPER, J.E. (1965) Epilepsy in a longitudinal survey of 5000 children. *Br. Med. J.*, **1**, 1020–1022.

CORBETT, J.A., TRIMBLE, M.R. and NICOL, T.C. (1985) Behavioural and cognitive impairments in children with epilepsy: The long term effects of anticonvulsant therapy. *J. Am. Acad. Child Psychiatry*, **24**, 17–23.

DHSS, DES and WELSH OFFICE (1976) *Fit for the Future: Report of the Committee of Child Health Services* chair S.D.M. COURT. HMSO, London.

ELLENBERG, J.H., HIRTZ, D.G. and NELSON, K.B. (1986) Do seizures in children cause intellectual deterioration? *N. Engl. J. Med.*, **314**, 1085–1088.

GREEN, S.H. (1987) Who needs a brain scan? *Arch. Dis. Child.*, 1094–1096.

GUDMUNDSSON, G. (1966) Epilepsy in Iceland. *Acta Neurol. Scand.*, **43** (suppl.), 25.

HOLDSWORTH, L. and WHITMORE, K. (1974) A study of children with epilepsy attending ordinary schools. 1: Their seizure patterns, progress and behaviour in school. *Dev. Med. Child Neurol.*, **16**, 746–758.

KANGESU, E., McGOWAN, M.E.L. and EDEH, J. (1984) Management of epilepsy in schools. *Arch. Dis. Child.*, **59**, 45–47.

KURTZ, Z., TOOKEY, P. and ROSS, E. (1987) The epidemiology of epilepsy in childhood. In E. ROSS, D. CHADWICK and R. CRAWFORD (eds) *Epilepsy in Young People*. John Wiley, Chichester, pp. 13–21.

MORGAN, J. and KURTZ, Z. (1986) *Special Services for People with Epilepsy*, HMSO, London.

MILLER, D.L., WADSWORTH, J., DIAMOND, J. and ROSS, E.M. (1985) Pertussis vaccine and whooping cough as risk factors in acute neurological illness and death in young children. *Dev. Biol. Standard*, **61**, 389–394.

Report of the Working Group on Services for People with Epilepsy (1986) HMSO, London.

ROGER, J., DRAVET, C., BUREAU, M., DREIFUSS, F.E. and WOLF, P. (1985) *Epileptic Syndromes in Infancy, Childhood and Adolescence*. Libbey, London and Paris.

ROSS, E.M. (1975) A Bristol study of epilepsy in secondary school children. *MD Dissertation*, University of Bristol.

ROSS, E.M. and BOMMEN, M. (1983) An epilepsy clinic for children: analysis of a year's work. *Br. J. Clin. Prac.*, Supplement **27**. 105–108.

ROSS, E.M. and PECKHAM, C.S. (1983) Seizure disorder in the National Child Development Study. In *Research Progress in Epilepsy* (ed. F.C. ROSE). Pitman Medical, Tunbridge Wells, pp. 46–59.

ROSS, E.M., PECKHAM, C.S., WEST, P.B. and BUTLER, N.R. (1980) Epilepsy in childhood: findings from the National Child Development Study. *Br. Med. J.*, **1**, 207–210.

RUTTER, M., GRAHAM, P. and YULE, W. (1972) *A Neuropsychiatric Study in Childhood*. Spastics International Medical Publications. London.

SILLANPAA M. (1973) Social prognosis of children with epilepsy. *Acta Paediatr. Scand.*, **237** (suppl.)

VERITY, C.M. and ROSS, E.M. (1985) Longitudinal studies of children's epilepsy. In *Paediatric Perspectives in Epilepsy* (eds ROSS E.M. and REYNOLDS, E.). John Wiley, Chichester, pp. 133–140.

WILKINS, A. (1987) Photosensitive epilepsy and visual display units. In *Epilepsy in Young People* (eds ROSS, E.M., CHADWICK, D. and CRAWFORD, R.). John Wiley, Chichester, pp. 147–155.

ZIELINSKY J.J. (1982) Epidemiology. In *A Textbook of Epilepsy* (eds J. LAIDLAW and A. RICHENS). Churchill Livingstone, Edinburgh, pp. 16–33.

8

Cognitive function and behaviour in children

CHRISTINE A. CULL
The David Lewis Centre for Epilepsy, Warford, Cheshire

A diagnosis of seizure disorder typically raises a number of questions with regard to the effect on a child's well-being, including cognitive function and behaviour. In this chapter I shall be addressing these issues, as they relate to children of school age, and attempt to tease out those factors which may have some prognostic significance, as suggested by a review of the literature.

EPILEPSY AND COGNITIVE FUNCTION

The term 'cognitive function' is being used in this context in its broadest sense, that is, the ability to learn and to perceive and process environmental information.

Intellectual ability

Early studies of cognitive function in children with epilepsy provided little more than a descriptive account of intellectual ability (as assessed by various IQ tests) in different groups of these children. The data thus collected were often pessimistic, showing that the mean scores obtained were below the mean of the particular test employed (Fox, 1924; Zimmerman et al., 1951; Davies-Eysenck, 1952). These are supported by more recent uncontrolled surveys (Gregoriades, 1972; Sillanpaa, 1973).

Studies incorporating control groups of children with no known neurological disorder provide further evidence that, as a group, children with epilepsy obtain lower IQ scores (Dawson and Conn, 1929; Sullivan and Gahagan, 1935; Halstead, 1957; Beck, 1959; Schwartz and Dennerll, 1970; Black, 1974; Black,

1976; Mellor and Lowit, 1977; Epir et al., 1984; Farwell et al., 1985).

Further analysis of these data indicated that the distribution of IQ scores was also different from that of the normal population and control groups, in that there were larger numbers of children than would be expected in the below average ranges (Sullivan and Gahagan, 1935; Zimmerman et al., 1951; Davies-Eysenck, 1952; Henderson, 1953; Keith et al., 1955; Bagley, 1970; Gregoriades, 1972; Sillanpaa, 1973; Mellor, 1977; Farwell et al., 1985).

However, there are also reports of children with epilepsy having normal (Bagley, 1970; Bourgeois et al., 1983) or higher than average mean scores on IQ tests (Collins and Lennox, 1947) which is not significantly different from control groups (Halstead, 1957; Heijbel and Bohman, 1975; Ellenberg et al., 1986) or their own siblings (Bourgeois et al., 1983; Ellenberg et al., 1986) supporting the notion that a seizure disorder can be compatible with the normal range of intellectual abilities.

Recently, attention has been drawn to the fact that IQ levels can fluctuate markedly in children with a seizure disorder. It is, therefore, important to bear in mind that, with respect to prognosis, a single assessment may be misleading, and a more reliable pattern of ability will be shown on repeated testing (Bourgeois et al., 1983; Rodin et al., 1986).

Scholastic performance and attainments

Real-life measures of cognitive function are few and, in children, the closest we have come is the use of attainment tests and other measures of school performance. Uncontrolled studies offer evidence that poor scholastic ability is common in children with epilepsy, even for those at normal schools (Fox, 1924; Rodin, 1968; Rodin et al., 1972; Holdsworth and Whitmore, 1974; Pazzaglia and Frank-Pazzaglia, 1976; Stedman et al., 1982; Farwell et al., 1985) whose performance is also worse than that expected on the basis of age and IQ (Seidenberg et al., 1986).

These findings are supported by controlled studies which demonstrate that the number of children with epilepsy who experience difficulties at school is significantly greater than in their non-epileptic peers (Rutter et al., 1970; Ross, 1973; Ross and West, 1978). This remains the case for a significant proportion of children even when IQ is taken into account (Green and Hartlage, 1971). On the other hand, their performance is no worse than that of children with learning problems (Black, 1976) or of behaviourally disturbed children (Bagley, 1971).

Impaired performance is seen particularly on tests of reading, spelling, arithmetic (Halstead, 1957; Rutter et al., 1970; Green and Hartlage, 1971; Ross, 1973; Ross and West, 1978; Stedman et al., 1982; Seidenberg et al., 1986) and word recognition (Seidenberg et al., 1986), but not on design copying (Ross and West, 1978) or tests of a creative rather than academic orientation (Ross, 1973).

Using a questionnaire approach, Bennett-Levy and Stores (1984) reported that teachers perceived children with epilepsy as being significantly worse than their non-epileptic peers with respect to attainments, alertness, concentration and the mental processing of information. When the level of attainment was controlled for, children with epilepsy were still perceived as being significantly less alert.

Other aspects of cognitive function

There is also evidence of impairments in more specific cognitive functions. On tests of visuomotor coordination, normal control groups were found to make significantly less errors than children with epilepsy (Beck, 1959; Tymchuck, 1974; Heijbel and Bohman, 1975) and to be quicker (Schwartz and Dennerll, 1970) even than those with idiopathic epilepsy (Shaw and Cruickshank, 1956). Poor performances have been reported on tests of psychomotor function, even in the presence of a normal IQ (Fox, 1924; Halstead, 1957). Visuoperceptual functions are also impaired (Morgan and Groh, 1980) although children with epilepsy are not significantly different from those with learning problems in this respect (Black, 1976). By contrast, no differences with respect to memory functions have been reported in comparison with matched control groups (Davies-Eysenck, 1952; Epir et al., 1984).

It may be that specific deficits in these areas contribute to difficulties at school experienced by some children with epilepsy in the presence of good intellectual functioning.

Factors affecting cognitive function

However, this is not the whole story. It is apparent to the clinician that children with epilepsy do not form a homogeneous group, but differ along a number of dimensions, namely aetiology; seizure variables (type, frequency, age of onset and duration of the seizure disorder); EEG activity; antiepileptic medication; sex and environment. Thus, it is important to raise the question as to the nature of the relationship between these variables and intellectual ability and scholastic performance. This may also help in understanding first, the discrepant findings with respect to intellectual ability; and secondly, the poor scholastic performance of children who are of at least average intellectual ability.

Aetiology

Aetiologically, there are two groups of epilepsies. The 'idiopathic' or 'uncomplicated' epileptics, where no cause can be established, and 'symptomatic' epilepsies which are associated with organic pathology or complicated by other neurological problems.

When children with epilepsy are compared with respect to this variable, those with symptomatic epilepsy are clearly at a disadvantage. Their IQ scores are significantly lower than those of children with idiopathic epilepsy (Collins and Lennox, 1947; Zimmerman et al., 1951; Halstead, 1957; Ounstead et al., 1966; Bourgeois et al., 1983), and there is a greater percentage of IQ scores within the handicap ranges (Price et al., 1948; Keith et al., 1955; Ounsted et al., 1966; Mellor, 1977). Conversely, children with idiopathic epilepsies are more likely to conform to the expected normal distribution for intellectual ability (Collins and Lennox, 1947; Price et al., 1948; Ounsted et al., 1966; Rutter et al., 1970).

Such a pattern of performance would also seem to be reflected in educational achievement (Halstead, 1957; Rodin, 1968).

As a corollary to this, Ellenberg et al. (1984) have presented evidence that neurological status within the first year of life, prior to the first seizure, may be an important prognostic indicator with respect to intellectual ability at seven years of age.

Thus, an organic aetiology for the seizures or a seizure disorder complicated by further neurological problems would appear to be a poor prognostic indicator for intellectual ability and scholastic performance.

Seizure variables

Seizure type. The relationship between seizure type and intellectual ability is unclear. Some studies have shown that petit mal seizures are commensurate with normal levels of intelligence, and that these children are less likely to be retarded (Collins and Lennox, 1947; Kaye, 1951; Zimmerman et al., 1951; Gregoriades, 1972; Sillanpaa, 1973), similarly for absence seizures (Bourgeois et al., 1983; Farwell et al., 1985). However, other investigators have found no relationship between petit mal seizures and IQ (Halstead, 1957). Children with grand mal seizures (Halstead, 1957), psychomotor or partial seizures have also been found to be unimpaired on tests of intellectual ability (Collins and Lennox, 1947; Sillanpaa, 1973; Whitehouse, 1975/76).

Major seizures have been reported to have a detrimental influence on intellectual ability (Sullivan and Gahagan, 1935; Henderson, 1953). Similarly, minor motor seizures and atypical absences may be associated with lower IQ values (Ellenberg et al., 1984; Farwell et al., 1985).

In a direct comparison of different seizure types, Giordani et al. (1985) found that children with partial seizures obtained better scores on some Wechsler subtests than did those with generalized or secondary generalized seizures, but there was no difference between these latter two groups.

Some studies have found no difference in the degree of retardation with respect to seizure type (Keith et al., 1955), whereas other investigators find that it is the number of different seizure types experienced that is important (Collins and Lennox, 1947; Schwartz and Dennerll, 1970; Mellor, 1970; Bourgeois et al., 1983).

Little in the way of a clear relationship between seizure type and poor attainments or educational underachievement has been reported (Bagley, 1970; Hartledge and Green, 1972), although major seizures have been implicated (Holdsworth and Whitmore, 1974) but focal seizures have not (Rodin, 1968).

Age of onset. By contrast, an early age of onset of the seizure disorder has more consistently been associated with lower IQ values (Sullivan and Gahagan, 1935; Collins and Lennox, 1947; Zimmerman et al., 1951; Keith et al., 1955; Ounsted et al., 1966; Sillanpaa, 1973; Mellor, 1977; Farwell et al., 1985) later onset conveying a positive prognosis for IQ (Kriz, 1978). This relationship would seem to hold true for both idiopathic (Zimmerman et al., 1951; Keith et al., 1955) and symptomatic epilepsies (Keith et al., 1955).

A long duration of seizure disorder has been negatively associated with IQ in three studies (Glaser, 1967; Bagley, 1971; Sillanpaa, 1973), with no association being found in a further study (Collins and Lennox, 1947).

An early age of onset and longstanding duration of epilepsy have also been implicated in learning difficulties (Rodin, 1968).

Seizure frequency. With respect to seizure frequency, the evidence would support the thesis that frequent seizures may have a detrimental effect on IQ (Henderson, 1953; Keith et al., 1955; Mazurowa, 1977; Ross and West, 1978; Niemann et al., 1985), for both idiopathic (Keith et al., 1955) and symptomatic epilepsies (Keith et al., 1955; Mazurowa 1977). The degree of seizure control would also seem to be important, good control being associated with higher IQ values (Farwell et al., 1985). But again, there are conflicting reports (Halstead, 1957). However, the number of studies is small and further evaluation of the effect of seizure frequency is needed.

It would seem that attainments and learning patterns are not related to seizure frequency (Rodin, 1968; Bagley, 1970; Hartlage and Green, 1972), although, again, seizure control may be important (Ross and Peckham, 1983).

EEG

An abnormal EEG would seem to be associated with a low IQ (Keith et al., 1955; Annett et al., 1961; Bagley, 1971), with the possible exception of the 3 cps spike and wave abnormality (Collins and Lennox, 1947; Bagley, 1971; Mellor, 1977) and Rolandic discharges (Heijbel and Bohman, 1975).

No clear relationship has been established with respect to attainments and school performance. However, memory functions may be impaired by temporal lobe abnormalities (Fedio and Mirskey, 1969), and generalized abnormalities may affect visuomotor coordination (Heijbel and Bohman, 1975) and sustained attention (Fedio and Mirskey, 1969; Stores, 1978). In addition, the occurrence of subclinical electric paroxysms can impair ongoing performance

(Davidoff and Johnson, 1964; Hutt, 1972; Hutt et al., 1977).

Antiepileptic medication

The reports available concerning antiepileptic medication are conflicting. Phenobarbitone (Ozdirim et al., 1978; Hellstrom and Barlach-Christoffersen, 1980), primidone (Nolte et al., 1980; Trimble and Corbett, 1980), phenytoin (Vallarta et al., 1974; Stores and Hart, 1976; Stores et al., 1978; Nolte et al., 1980; Trimble and Corbett, 1980), ethosuximide (Guey et al., 1967; Roger et al., 1968), sodium valproate (Trimble and Corbett, 1980) and carbamazepine (Martin et al., 1965; Schain et al., 1981) have all been reported to lead to detrimental effects.

Beneficial effects have been found for ethosuximide (Browne et al., 1975), sodium valproate (Barnes and Bower, 1975; Harding et al., 1980) and carbamazepine (Martin et al., 1965; Rett, 1976; Schain et al., 1977; Jacobides, 1978).

However, it is not just the drug used that is of importance, the way it is used must also be considered. In studies we have carried out at Queen Square and Great Ormond Street, children with epilepsy assessed on a variety of automated tests demonstrated an improvement in cognitive functioning following a decrease in drug dose, but no improvement was seen for children undergoing an increase. It also seemed that children on polytherapy regimens were at more of a disadvantage than those on monotherapy.

Sex

The findings with respect to sex and intellectual ability are conflicting. Early studies report a superiority for boys (Fox, 1924; Halstead, 1957) or no difference (Keith et al., 1955), whereas others have found girls to be superior (Sullivan and Gahagan, 1935; Schwartz and Dennerll, 1970; Mellor and Lowit, 1977).

There is however, some suggestion that boys are more likely to underachieve at school (Holdsworth and Whitmore, 1974), and to be impaired with respect to reading skills (Stores and Hart, 1976; Stedman et al., 1982). But again there are some conflicting findings, Seidenberg et al. (1986) finding no significant sex effect with respect to underachievement on a number of attainment tests.

Family and environmental influence

Environmental factors have received scant attention in the epilepsy literature. The few available studies suggest that parental attitudes and the reactions of a child's peers can influence the academic attainment and school performance of the child with epilepsy, (Bagley, 1970; Hartlage and Green, 1972; Pazzaglia and Frank-Pazzaglia, 1976; Long and Moore, 1979).

EPILEPSY AND BEHAVIOUR

Prevalence of behaviour disorder

Surveys of the prevalence of behavioural problems in children with epilepsy suggest that 12–95% exhibit some form of disturbance. The estimates vary according to the population studied. They are lowest in normal population samples, such as in normal schools or general practice, being somewhere in the region of 12–23% (Henderson, 1953; Pond and Bidwell, 1959; Holdsworth and Whitmore, 1974). This figure rises to about 50% of those attending outpatient epilepsy clinics (Price et al., 1948; Rodin, 1968), and can be as high as 95% in children requiring specialist inpatient treatment (Stores, 1982).

In controlled studies, children with epilepsy are found to have a significantly greater occurrence of behaviour disturbance than those without epilepsy (Rutter et al., 1970; Bagley, 1971; Mellor et al., 1974; Hackney and Taylor, 1976; Stores, 1977; Hoare, 1984a; Epir et al., 1984), including their own siblings (Richardson and Friedman, 1974; Long and Moore, 1979; Epir et al., 1984), and children with other chronic disorders (Hoare, 1984a). But they are no different from others with organic pathology (Beck, 1959) and psychiatric clinic attenders (Hackney and Taylor, 1976). However, it is important to note that some investigators have reported that children with epilepsy attending ordinary schools are no different from their peers in this respect (Heijbl and Bohman, 1975; Ross and West, 1978; Ross and Peckham, 1983).

In spite of this, the majority of studies suggest that children with epilepsy are at risk for developing behaviour disorders, and the factors that may contribute to that risk will now be discussed.

Factors affecting behaviour

Aetiology

The relationship between aetiology and behaviour disturbance has been poorly investigated. Evidence of organic pathology has been reported for the majority of children exhibiting behaviour disorders (Sillanpaa, 1973) and large numbers of children with behaviour disorders have been found in brain-damaged populations (Mazurowa, 1977). There are more children with brain damage in behaviour-disordered groups than children without brain damage (Bagley, 1971) and there is a greater but nonsignificant incidence of behaviour disorder in children with complicated as opposed to uncomplicated epilepsy (Rutter et al., 1970).

In addition, children who perform poorly on neuropsychological measures have been reported to manifest significantly more psychopathology and aggression than those with good neuropsychological functioning, and to be less socially competent (Hermann, 1982).

Thus, the little available evidence shows only trends in the direction of an association between organic aetiology and behaviour disturbance.

Epilepsy variables

Seizure type. The relationship between behaviour disturbance and seizure type is even less clear. An increased occurrence of behaviour disorder has been found to be associated with focal seizures (Rodin, 1968), temporal lobe epilepsy (Rutter et al., 1970; Gregoriades, 1972); complex partial seizures (Hoare, 1984a); major seizures (Henderson, 1953; Holdsworth and Whitmore, 1974); grand mal seizures (Pazzaglia and Frank-Pazzaglia, 1976); and petit mal seizures (Halstead, 1957). It has also been suggested that the number of different seizure types may be an important factor (Mellor, 1977). Hermann et al. (1981) compared children with temporal lobe seizures, primary generalized and focal nontemporal seizures, and found no difference with respect to the occurrence of behaviour disorder. However, the focal nontemporal group obtained a significantly lower score on a measure of aggression than those with temporal lobe seizures. In a further study, no differences were found between temporal lobe and primary generalized seizures (Whitmore et al., 1982).

Age of onset. Again investigations of the role of age of onset are few and the findings contradictory, but they suggest a trend towards increased rates of behaviour disturbance with early age of onset (Sullivan and Gahagan, 1935; Ounsted et al., 1966; Rodin, 1968), although a lack of association has also been reported (Rutter et al., 1970). Similarly, there are conflicting reports concerning the role of duration of the seizure disorder (Pazzaglia and Frank-Pazzaglia, 1976; Hoare, 1984a).

Seizure frequency. Positive associations between seizure frequency and behaviour disturbance have been reported in some studies (Halstead, 1957; Holdsworth and Whitmore, 1974; Hoare, 1984a) and no association in others (Henderson, 1953; Rutter et al., 1970).

EEG

Some studies have found no relationship between an abnormal EEG and behaviour disturbance (Hartlage et al., 1972; Mellor, 1977). However, in other investigations, a temporal lobe focus has been found to be associated with disturbed behaviour (Stores, 1977; Whitman et al., 1982; Hoare, 1984a), and with aggressive behaviour (Bagley, 1973) and dependency (Stores and Piran, 1978).

Antiepileptic medication

Phenobarbitone (Ingram, 1956; Ozdirim et al., 1978), phenytoin (Patel and Chrichton, 1968; Vallarta et al., 1974) and sodium valproate (Barnes and Bower, 1975; Egger and Brett, 1981) have all been implicated in behavioural disturbance. However, sodium valproate has also been suggested to exert no significant effect on behaviour (Sonnen et al., 1975; Herranz et al., 1982), and beneficial effects have been reported for phenytoin (Merritt and Putnam, 1938; Ozdirim et al., 1978). Carbamazepine has been associated with considerable improvements in behaviour (Donner and Frisk, 1975; Jacobides, 1978); however, a small number of children may show idiosyncratic negative reactions (Silverstein et al., 1982). Clobazam may also be beneficial (Gastaut, 1981).

In studies with Dr Trimble and Dr John Wilson, we found that improvements in behaviour (as assessed by a questionnaire completed by parents) were associated with a reduction in antiepileptic drug load, whereas children whose medication load was being increased failed to show such changes. However, there were no significant differences in behaviour questionnaire scores for children on polytherapy and monotherapy regimens.

Sex

No significant difference between the number of boys and girls exhibiting behaviour disturbance has been reported in some studies (Halstead, 1957; Rutter et al., 1970; Holdsworth and Whitmore, 1974). However, there are also reports of a greater number of disturbed boys relative to girls with epilepsy (Sullivan and Gahagan, 1935; Henderson, 1953; Pond and Bidwell, 1959/60; Ounsted et al., 1966; Mellor, 1977; Whitman et al., 1982) and nonepileptic boys (Stores, 1977). More specifically, it has been suggested that any gender bias depends upon the type of behaviour disturbance. Thus aggressive, anti-social behaviour disorders have been associated with boys (Bagley, 1973; Hackney and Taylor, 1976; Mellor, 1977) whereas neurotic disturbances are found more frequently in girls (Hackney and Taylor, 1976; Mellor, 1977).

Family and environmental influences

A wide range of family and environmental influences has been implicated in the development of behaviour disorders, in uncontrolled studies as follows: a disturbed home and family discord (Pond and Bidwell, 1959/60; Ounsted et al., 1966); maladaptive or negative family and parental attitudes (Price et al., 1948;

Pond and Bidwell, 1954; Hartlage and Green, 1972); overanxious parents (Bidwell, 1952); inappropriate child management (Stores, 1982), and parental disturbance (Rutter et al., 1970). In controlled studies, similar factors were found to discriminate between disturbed and nondisturbed children with epilepsy (Grunberg and Pond, 1957; Bagley, 1971; Hoare, 1984b).

BEHAVIOUR AND COGNITIVE FUNCTION

There seems to be a clear link between poor cognitive function and behaviour disturbance. Thus low IQs are more likely to be associated with behaviour disorder (Halstead, 1957; Sillanpaa, 1973; Mellor and Lowit, 1977), and vice versa (Henderson, 1953; Rutter et al., 1970; Mellor, 1977), similarly for poor school performance (Halstead, 1957; Rodin, 1968; Holdsworth and Whitmore, 1974; Pazzaglia and Frank-Pazzaglia, 1976). However, it would seem that children who perform poorly on attainment tests are not necessarily disturbed (Bagley, 1971; Stores and Hart, 1976), whereas children who are behaviourally disturbed are more likely to be underachieving (Rutter et al., 1970; Holdsworth and Whitmore, 1974).

CONCLUSION

Thus, it can be tentatively concluded that intellectual ability may be influenced by the presence of brain damage, factors related to the epilepsy itself and an abnormal EEG, and may be exacerbated by anti-epileptic medication.

Poor attainments and scholastic ability are accounted for in part by a low IQ, but there remains a significant number of children of good intellectual ability who are underachieving. No clear association with seizure variables has been established, although seizure type, frequency, age of onset and duration of the seizure disorder have all been implicated. The relationship with interictal EEG abnormality has yet to be clarified, whereas the occurrence of subclinical bursts of electrical activity has been found to impair ongoing performance. Boys seem to be disadvantaged and parental attitudes are an important, though little investigated, influence. In addition, learning problems may be due to specific cognitive deficits in the areas of visuomotor coordination, visuoperceptual functioning, psychomotor ability, and lowered alertness.

Aetiology, factors related to the epilepsy itself, EEG abnormality, gender and medication, may all have a role to play in the genesis of behaviour disorder; however, the nature of this association requires further clarification. In contrast, adverse familial and environmental factors are clearly an important contributory factor.

REFERENCES

ANNETT, M., LEE, D. and OUNSTED, C. (1961) Intellectual disabilities in relation to lateralised features in the EEG. In *Hemiplegic Cerebral Palsy in Children and Adults*. Little Club Clinics in Developmental Medicine, No. 4.

BAGLEY, C. (1970) The educational performance of children with epilepsy. *Brit. J. Educational Psychol.,* **40**, 82–83.

BAGLEY, C. (1971) *The Social Psychology of the Child with Epilepsy*. Routledge and Kegan Paul, London.

BAGLEY, C. (1973) Multiple influences on deviant behaviour in children with epilepsy. *J. Biosocial Sci.,* **5**, 1–16.

BARNES, S.E. and BOWER, B.D. (1975) Sodium valproate in the treatment of intractable childhood epilepsy. *Dev. Med. Child Neurol.,* **17**, 175–181.

BECK, H.S. (1959) Comparison of convulsive organic, non-convulsive organic, and non-organic public school children. *Am. J. Ment. Defic.,* **63**, 866–875.

BENNETT-LEVY, J. and STORES, G. (1984) The nature of cognitive dysfunction in school-children with epilepsy. *Acta Neurol. Scand.,* **69**, Suppl. 99, 79–82.

BIDWELL, B. (1952) Problems of families with epileptic children. *Mental Health (London),* **11**, 104–110.

BLACK, F.W. (1974) Patterns of cognitive impairment in children with suspected and documented neurological dysfunction. *Percep. Motor Skills,* **39**, 115–120.

BLACK, F.W. (1976) Learning problems and seizure disorders. *J. Pediat. Psychol.,* 32–34.

BOURGEOIS, B.F.D., PRENSKY, A.L., PALKES, H.S., TALENT, B.K. and BUSCH, S.G. (1983) Intelligence in epilepsy: a prospective study in children. *Ann. Neurol.,* **14**, 438–444.

BROWNE, T.R., DREIFUSS, F.E., DYKEN, P.R., GOODE, D.J., PENRY, J.K., PORTER, R.J., WHITE, B.G. and WHITE, P.T. (1975) Ethosuximide in the treatment of absence (petit mal) seizures. *Neurology,* **25**, 515–524.

COLLINS, A.L. and LENNOX, W.G. (1947) The intelligence of 300 private epileptic patients. *Research Publications Association for Research in Nervous and Mental Disease,* **XXVI** 586–603.

DAVIDOFF, R.A. and JOHNSON, L.C. (1964) Paroxysmal EEC activity and cognitive-motor performance. *Electroenceph. Clin. Neurophysiol.,* **16**, 343–354.

DAVIES-EYSENCK, M. (1952) Cognitive factors in epilepsy *J. Neurol., Neurosurg. Psychiat.,* **15**, 39–44.

DAWSON, S. and CONN, J.C.M. (1929) The intelligence of epileptic children. *Arch. Dis. Child.,* **4**, 142–151.

DONNER, M. and FRISK, M. (1965) Carbamazepine treatment of epileptic and psychic symptoms in children and adolescents. *Ann. Paediatria Fenniae,* **11**, 91–97.

EGGER, J. and BRETT, E.M. (1981) Effects of sodium valproate in 100 children with special reference to weight. *Br. Med. J.,* **283**, 577–581.

ELLENBERG, J.H., HIRTZ, D.G. and NELSON, K.B. (1984) Age at onset of seizures in young children. *Ann. Neurol.,* **15**, 127–134.

ELLENBERG, J.H., HIRTZ, D.G. and NELSON, K.B. (1986) Do seizures in children cause intellectual deterioration? *N. Engl. J. Med.,* **314**, 1085–1088.

EPIR, S., RENDA, Y. and BASER, N. (1984) Cognitive and behavioural characteristics of children with idiopathic epilepsy in a low-income area of Ankara, Turkey. *Dev. Med. Child Neurol.,* **26**, 200–207.

FARWELL, J.R., DODRILL, C.B. and MATZEL, L.W. (1985) Neuropsychological abilities of children with epilepsy. *Epilepsia,* **26**, 395–400.

FEDIO, P. and MIRSKY, A.F. (1969) Selective intellectual deficits in children with temporal lobe or centrencephalic epilepsy. *Neuropsychologia,* **7**, 287–300.

FOX, J.T. (1924) The response of epileptic children to mental and educational tests. *Brit. J. Med. Psychol.,* **4**, 235–248.

GASTAUT, H. (1981) The effect of benzodiazepines on chronic epilepsy in man (with particular reference to clobazam). In *Clobazam: The Royal Society of Medicine International Congress and Symposium Series, Number 43*, (eds I. HINDMARCH and P.D. STONIER), pp. 141–150. The Royal Society of Medicine, Academic Press, London.

GIORDANI, B., BERENT, S., SACKELLARES, J.C., ROURKE, D., SEIDENBERG, M., O'LEARY, D.S., DREIFUSS, F.E. and BOLL, T.J. (1985) Intelligence test performance of patients with partial and generalised seizures. *Epilepsia*, **26**, 37–42.

GLASER, G.H. (1967) Limbic epilepsy in childhood. *J. Nerv. Ment. Dis.*, **144**, 391–397.

GREEN, J.B. and HARTLAGE, L.C. (1971) Comparative performance of epileptic and non epileptic children and adolescents. *Dis. Nerv. Sys.*, **32**, 418–421.

GREGORIADES, A.D. (1972) A medical and social survey of 231 children with seizures. *Epilepsia*, **13**, 13–20.

GRUNBERG, F. and POND, D.A. (1957) Conduct disorders in epileptic children. *J. Neurol., Neurosurg., Psychiat.*, **20**, 65–68.

GUEY, J., CHARLES, C., COQUERY, C., ROGER, J. and SOULAYROL, R. (1967) Study of psychological effects of ethosuximide (Zarontin) on 25 children suffering from petit male epilepsy. *Epilepsia*, **8**, 129–141.

HACKNEY, A. and TAYLOR, D.C. (1976) A teacher's questionnaire description of epileptic children. *Epilepsia*, **17**, 175–281.

HALSTEAD, H. (1957) Abilities and behaviour of epileptic children. *J. Ment. Sci.*, **103**, 28–47.

HARDING, G.F.A., PULLAN, J.J. and DRASDO, N. (1980) The effect of sodium valproate and other anticonvulsants on performance in children and adolescents. In *The Place of Sodium Valproate in the Treatment of Epilepsy: The Royal Society of Medicine International Congress and Symposium Series, Number 30* (eds M.J. PARSONAGE and A.D.S. CALDWELL), pp. 61–71. The Royal Society of Medicine, Academic Press, Grune & Stratton, London.

HARTLAGE, L.C. and GREEN, J.B. (1972) The relation of parental attitudes to academic and social achievement in epileptic children. *Epilepsia*, **13**, 21–26.

HARTLAGE, L.C., GREEN, J.B. and OFFUTT, L. (1972) Dependency in epileptic children. *Epilepsia*, **13**, 27–30.

HEIJBEL, J. and BOHMAN, M. (1975) Benign epilepsy of children with centrotemporal EEG foci: intelligence, behaviour, and school adjustment. *Epilepsia*, **16**, 679–687.

HELLSTROM, B. and BARLACH-CHRISTOFFERSEN, M. (1980) Influence of phenobarbital on the psychomotor development and behaviour in preschool children with convulsions. *Neuropaediatrie*, **11**, 151–160.

HENDERSON, P. (1953) Epilepsy in school children, *Brit. J. Prevent. Social Med.*, **7**, 9–13.

HERMANN, B.P. (1982) Neuropsychological functioning and psychopathology in children with epilepsy. *Epilepsia*, **23**, 545–554.

HERMANN, B.P., BLACK, R.B. and CHHABRIA, S. (1981) Behavioural problems and social competence in children with epilepsy. *Epilepsia*, **22**, 703–710.

HERRANZ, J.L., ARTEAGA, R. and ARMIJO, J.A. (1982) Side effects of sodium valproate in monotherapy controlled by plasma levels: a study of 88 pediatric patients. *Epilepsia*, **23**, 203–214.

HOARE, P. (1984a) The development of psychiatric disorder among schoolchildren with epilepsy, *Dev. Med. Child Neurol.*, **26**, 3–13.

HOARE, P. (1984b) Does illness foster dependency? A study of epileptic and diabetic children. *Dev. Med. Child Neurol.*, **26**, 20–24.

HOLDSWORTH, L. and WHITMORE, K. (1974) A study of children with epilepsy attending ordinary schools. I: Their seizure patterns, prognosis and behaviour in school. *Dev. Med. Child Neurol.*, **16**, 746–758.

HUTT, S.J. (1972) Experimental analysis of brain activity and behaviour in children with 'minor' seizures. *Epilepsia*, **13**, 520–534.

HUTT, S.J., NEWTON, J. and FAIRWEATHER, H. (1977) Choice reaction time and EEG activity in children with epilepsy. *Neuropsychologia*, **15**, 257–267.

INGRAM, T.T.S. (1956) A characteristic form of overactive behaviour in brain damaged children. *J. Ment. Sci.*, **102**, 550–558.

JACOBIDES, G.M. (1978) Alertness and scholastic achievement in young epileptics treated with carbamazepine (Tegretol). In *Advances in Epileptology – 1977* (eds, H. MEINARDI and A.J. ROWAN), pp. 114–119. Swets & Zeitlinger B.V., Amsterdam.

KAYE, I. (1951) What are the evidences of social and psychological maladjustment revealed in a study of seventeen children who have idiopathic petit mal epilepsy? *J. Child Psychiat.*, **2**, 115–160.

KEITH, H.M., EWERT, J.C., GREEN, M.W. and GAGE, R.P. (1955) Mental status of children with convulsive disorders. *Neurology*, **5**, 419–425.

KRIZ, M. (1978) Epilepsy in older school children. In *Advances in Epileptology – 1977* (eds H. MEINARDI and A.J. ROWAN), pp. 38–41. Swets & Zeitlinger B.V., Amsterdam.

LONG, C.G. and MOORE, J.R. (1979) Parental expectations for their epileptic children. *J. Child Psychol. and Psychiat.*, **20**, 299–312.

MARTIN, F., MOVARREKHI, M. and GISIGER, M.G. (1965) Etude de quelques effets du tegretol sur une population d'enfants épileptiques. *Schweiz. Medizin. Wochen.*, **95**, 992–989.

MAZUROWA, M. (1977) Psychological evaluation of children with post traumatic epilepsy (catamnestic examinations). In *Posttraumatic Epilepsy and Pharmacological Prophylaxis* (ed J. MAJKOWSKI), pp. 69–73. Polish Chapter of the International League Against Epilepsy, Warszawa.

MELLOR, D.H. (1977) A study of epilepsy in childhood with particular reference to behaviour disorder. MD Thesis, University of Leeds.

MELLOR, D.H. and LOWIT, I. (1977) A study of intellectual function in children with epilepsy attending ordinary schools. In *Epilepsy, The Eighth International Symposium* (ed. J.K. PENRY), pp. 291–294. Raven Press, New York.

MELLOR, D.H., LOWIT, I. and HALL, D.J. (1974) Are epileptic children behaviourally different from other children? In *Epilepsy: Proceedings of the Hans Berger Centenary Symposium* (eds P. HARRIS and C. MAWDSLEY), pp. 313–316. Churchill-Livingstone, Edinburgh.

MERRITT, H.H. and PUTNAM, T.J. (1938) Sodium diphenyl hydantoinate in the treatment of convulsive disorders. *J. Am. Med. Ass.*, **111**, 1068–1073.

MORGAN, A.M.B. and GROH, C. (1980) Visual perceptual deficits in young children with epilepsy. In *Epilepsy and Behaviour '79* (eds B. KULIG, H. MEINARDI and G. STORES), pp. 169–171. Swets & Zeitlinger B.V., Lisse.

NIEMANN, H., BOENICK, H.E., SCHMIDT, R.C. and ETTLINGER, G. (1985) Cognitive development in epilepsy: the relative influence of epileptic activity and of brain damage. *European Archives of Psychiatry and Neurological Sciences*, **234**, 399–403.

NOLTE, R., WETZEL, B., BRUGMANN, G. and BRINTZINGER, I. (1980) Effects of phenytoin- and primidone-monotherapy on mental performance in children. In *Antiepileptic Therapy: Advances in Drug Monitoring* (eds S.I. JOHANNESSEN, P.L. MORSELLI, C.E. PIPPENGER, A. RICHENS, D. SCHMIDT and H. MEINARDI), pp. 81–86. Raven Press, New York.

OUNSTED, C., LINDSAY, J. and NORMAN, R. (1966) Biological factors in temporal lobe epilepsy. *Clinics in Developmental Medicine*, No. 22. Spastics Society Medical Education and Information Unit, Heinemann Medical Books, London.

OZDIRIM, E., RENDA, Y. and EPIR, S. (1978) Effects of phenobarbital and phentoin on the behaviour of epileptic children. In *Advances in Epileptology – 1977* (eds H. MEINARDI and A.J. ROWAN), pp. 120–123. Swets & Zeitlinger B.V., Amsterdam.

PATEL, H. and CHRICHTON, J.U. (1968) The neurologic hazards of diphenylhydantoin in childhood. *J. Pediat.*, **73**, 676–684.

PAZZAGLIA, P. and FRANK-PAZZAGLIA, L. (1976) Record in grade school of pupils with epilepsy: an epidemiological study. *Epilepsia*, **17**, 361–366.

POND, D.A. and BIDWELL, B. (1954) Management of behaviour disorders in epileptic children. *Brit. Med. J.*, **II**, 1520–1523.

POND, D.A. and BIDWELL, B.H. (1959/60) A survey of epilepsy in fourteen general practices. II. Social and psychological aspects. *Epilepsia*, **1**, 285–299.

PRICE, J.C., KOGAN, K.L. and TOMPKINS, L.R. (1948) The prevalence and incidence of extramural epilepsy. In *Epilepsy: Psychiatric Aspects of Convulsive Disorders* (eds P.M. HOCH and R.P. KNIGHT), pp. 48–57. William Heinemann, Medical Books, London.

RETT, A. (1976) The so-called psychotropic effect of Tegretol in the treatment of convulsions of cerebral origin in children. In *Epileptic Seizures – Behaviour – Pain*. Ed. W. BIRKMAYER, pp. 194–204. Hans Huber Publishers, Bern.

RICHARDSON, D.W. and FRIEDMAN, S.B. (1974) Psychosocial problems of the adolescent patient with epilepsy. *Clin. Pediat.*, 121–126.

RODIN, E.A. (1968) *The Prognosis of Patients with Epilepsy*. Charles C. Thomas, Springfield, USA.

RODIN, E., RENNICK, P., DENNERLL, R. and LIN, Y. (1972) Vocational and educational problems of epileptic patients. *Epilepsia*, **13**, 149–160.

RODIN, E.A., SCHMALTZ, S. and TWITTY, G. (1986) Intellectual function of patients with childhood epilepsy. *Dev. Med. & Child Neurol.*, **28**, 25–33.

ROGER, J., GRAGEON, H., GUEY, J. and LOB, H. (1968) Incidences psychiatriques et psychologiques du traitement par l'ethosuccimide chez les epileptiques. *L'Encephale*, **57**, 407–438.

ROSS, E.M. (1973) Convulsive disorders in British Children. *Proceedings of the Royal Society of Medicine*, **66**, 703–704.

ROSS, E.M. and PECKHAM, C.S. (1983) Schoolchildren with epilepsy. In *Advances in Epileptology: XIVth Epilepsy International Symposium* (eds M. PARSONAGE, R.H.E. GRANT, A.G. CRAIG and A.A. WARD Jr), pp. 215–220. Raven Press, New York.

ROSS, E.M. and WEST, P.B. (1978) Achievements and problems of British eleven year olds with epilepsy. In *Advances in Epileptology – 1977* (eds H. MEINARDI and A.J. ROWAN), pp. 34–37. Swets & Zeitlinger, B.V., Amsterdam.

RUTTER, M., GRAHAM, P. and YULE, W. (1970) A neuropsychiatric study in childhood. *Clinics in Developmental Medicine*, **35/36**. Published jointly by Spastics International Medical Publications and Heinemann Medical Books, London.

SCHAIN, R.J., WARD, J.W. and GUTHRIE, D. (1977) Carbamazepine as an anticonvulsant in children. *Neurology*, **27**, 476–480.

SCHAIN, R.J., SHIELDS, W.D. and DREISBACH, M. (1981) Comparison of carbamazepine and phenobarbital in treatment of children with epilepsy. Paper presented at the XIIIth Epilepsy International Symposium, Kyoto, Japan.

SCHWARTZ, M.L. and DENNERLL, R.D. (1970) Neuropsychological assessment of children with, without, and with questionable epileptogenic dysfunction. *Percep. Motor Skills*, **30**, 111–121.

SEIDENBERG, M., BECK, N., GEISSER, M., GIORDANI, B., SACKELLARES, J.C., BERENT, S., DREIFUSS, F.E. & BOLL, T.J. (1986) Academic achievement of children with epilepsy. *Epilepsia*, **27**, 753–759.

SHAW, M.C. and CRUICKSHANK, W.M. (1956) The use of the Bender Gestalt test with epileptic children. *J. Clin. Psychol.*, **12**, 192–193.

SILLANPAA, M. (1973) Medico-social prognosis of children with epilepsy: epidemiological study and analysis of 245 patients. *Acta Paed. Scand.*, Suppl. **237**, 3–104.

SILVERSTEIN, F.S., PARRISH, M.A. and JOHNSTON, M.V. (1982) Adverse behavioural reactions in children treated with carbamazepine (Tegretol). *J. Pediat.*, **101**, 785–787.

SONNEN, A.E.H., ZELVEDER, W.H. and BRUENS, J.H. (1975) A double blind study of the influence of dipropylacetate on behaviour. *Acta Neurol. Scand.*, Suppl. **60**, 43–47.

STEDMAN, J., VAN HEYNINGEN, R. and LINDSAY, J. (1982) Educational underachievement and epilepsy. A study of children from normal schools admitted to a special hospital for epilepsy. *Early Child Devel. Care*, **9**, 65–82.

STORES, G. (1977) Behaviour disturbance and type of epilepsy in children attending ordinary school. In *Epilepsy, The Eigth International Symposium*. (ed. J.K. PENRY), pp. 245–249. Raven Press, New York.

STORES, G. (1978) Sex-related differences in 'attentiveness' in children with epilepsy attending ordinary school. In *Advances in Epileptology – 1977* (eds H. MEINARDI and A.J. ROWAN), pp. 54–57. Swets & Zeitlinger B.V., Amsterdam.

STORES, G. (1982) Psychosocial preventive measures and rehabilitation of children with epilepsy. In *Advances in Epileptology: XIIIth Epilepsy International Symposium* (eds H. AKIMOTO, H. KAZAMATSURI, M. SEINO and A. WARD), pp. 437–439. Raven Press, New York.

STORES, G. and HART, J. (1976) Reading skills of children with generalised or focal epilepsy attending ordinary school. *Dev. Med. Child Neurol.*, **18**, 705–716.

STORES, G. and PIRAN, N. (1978) Dependency of different types in school children with epilepsy. *Psychol. Med.*, **8**, 441–445.

STORES, G., HART, J. and PIRAN, N. (1978) Inattentiveness in school children with epilepsy. *Epilepsia*, **19**, 169–175.

SULLIVAN, E.B. and GAHAGAN, L. (1935) On intelligence of epileptic children. *Genetic Psychology Monographs*, **XVII**, 309–376.

TRIMBLE, M.R. and CORBETT, J.A. (1980) Behavioural and cognitive disturbances in epileptic children. *Irish Med. J.*, **73**, Suppl. 10, 21–28.

TYMCHUK, A.J. (1974) Comparison of Bender error and time scores for groups of epileptic, retarded and behaviour-problem children. *Percep. Motor Skills*, **38**, 71–74.

VALLARTA, J.M., BELL, D.B. and REICHERT, A. (1974) Progressive encephalopathy due to chronic hydantoin intoxication. *Am. J. Dis. Child.*, **128**, 27–34.

WHITEHOUSE, D. (1975/76) Behaviour and learning problems in epileptic children. *Behav. Neuropsychiat.*, **7**, 23–29.

WHITMAN, S., HERMANN, B.P., BLACK, R.B. and CHHABRIA, S. (1982) Psychopathology and seizure type in children with epilepsy. *Psychol. Med.*, **12**, 843–853.

ZIMMERMAN, F.T., BURGEMEISTER, B.B. and PUTMAN, T.J. (1951) Intellectual and emotional makeup of the epileptic, *Arch. Neurol. Psychiat.*, **65**, 545–556.

9

Cognitive deterioration in children with epilepsy

F.M.C. BESAG
Lingfield Hospital School, Surrey

INTRODUCTION

Although Hippocrates in 400 BC expressed the view that the cause of 'the sacred disease' did not lie in the supernatural but in dysfunction of the brain, superstition and misconceptions about the natural course of epilepsy have continued. Aretaeus, the Cappadocian, AD 81–138, wrote,

> but if it becomes inveterate the patients are not free from harm even in the intervals, but are languid, spiritless, stupid, inhuman, unsociable, and not disposed to hold intercourse, nor to be sociable at any period of life, sleepless, subject to many horrid dreams, without appetite, and with bad digestion; pale, of leaden colours; slow to learn, from torpidity of the understanding and of the senses; dull of hearing; have noises and ringing in the head; utterance indistinct and bewildered, either from the nature of the disease, or from wounds during attacks; the tongue is rolled about the mouth convulsively in various ways. The disease also sometimes disturbs the understanding so that the patient becomes altogether fatuous.

William Gowers appeared to have no doubt about the link between epilepsy and deterioration when he wrote:

> The mental state of epileptics, as is well known, freqently presents deterioration. In its slighter forms there is merely defective memory. In more severe degree there is greater imperfection of intellectual power, weakened capacity for attention and often defective moral control. Mischievous restlessness and irritability in childhood may develop to vicious and even criminal tendencies in adult life. Every grade of intellect defect may be met with down to actual imbecility.

But he qualified this by adding:

> The mental state must not be regarded in all instances as entirely the effect of the
> disease. It is certainly, in some, the expression of a cerebral imperfection of which
> the epilepsy is another manifestation. In such instances mental defect exists
> before the occurrence of the first fit. In other cases, however, which constitute a
> majority of the whole, the failure must be regarded as a consequence of the
> disease. It distinctly succeeds the fits in point of time, and may lessen very much
> when the fits are arrested by treatment. It is not surprising, therefore, that in cases
> in which a mental defect exists before the fits commence, this should be greatly
> intensified by the subsequent attacks.

Systematic studies using sequential cognitive testing opened a new era in the
approach to the questions surrounding the possible link between epilepsy and
cognitive deterioration in children. One of the earliest studies using sequential
testing was carried out by J. Tylor Fox at Lingfield in 1924. The tradition of
studying the children in this establishment has been continued by Corbett et al.
(1985a) and by the present author. Some of the most recent data from Lingfield
Hospital School are presented in this chapter.

Despite the number of studies which have now been carried out, and
notwithstanding some excellent reviews, notably those by Brown and
Reynolds (1981), Addy (1987) and Lesser et al. (1986), certain fundamental
questions still create confusion because of the apparently conflicting answers to
them in the literature. A careful examination of research work carried out to
date enables some of these issues to be clarified and indicates what studies still
need to be performed.

A useful framework for examining these matters is provided by considering
the following questions. 1. Is epilepsy associated with deterioration? 2. Does
epilepsy cause deterioration? 3. Does deterioration cause epilepsy? 4. Do both
epilepsy and deterioration reflect some underlying causative brain abnormality? 5. When epilepsy and cognitive deterioration occur together, what factors
might be important?

IS EPILEPSY ASSOCIATED WITH DETERIORATION?

In 1924 J. Tylor Fox, the Medical Superintendent at Lingfield, carried out a
battery of 14 tests on 150 students in this residential school for children with
epilepsy. As part of this study, Binet tests were given to 130 children in two
successive years. Eight per cent of these children deteriorated by more than 10
points and only one child improved by more than 10 points. Cookson (1927)
examined 100 children with epilepsy and found 'marked mental deficiency' in
26. Dawson and Conn (1929) collected sequential IQ data on 21 children with
epilepsy. Sixteen deteriorated, five of these by more than 10 points. Three
children improved to a small degree which was not statistically significant and
two had a stationary IQ. Chaudhry and Pond (1961) compared a group of 28

children suffering with epilepsy who deteriorated with a control group of 28 who did not. This and other studies emphasized the fact that not all children with epilepsy deteriorate although there is marked deterioration in some.

Hung (1968) studied 500 patients with epilepsy in a mixed group of adults and children. About one quarter were found to have intellectual impairment. Many other studies have shown an association between intellectual impairment and epilepsy. Some of these refer to 'deterioration' without having carried out two or more tests of cognitive function over a period of time. It is assumed in a number of these accounts that because epilepsy and cognitive impairment are associated, their data indicate deterioration from normal ability has occurred. Pond and Bidwell (1960), in a study of 14 general practices, found that one third of the schoolage children with epilepsy had educational difficulties. Rutter et al. (1970), in the Isle of Wight study, found that almost one fifth of the children with epilepsy had substantially impaired reading abilities. Pazzaglia and Frank-Pazzaglia (1976) surveyed 13,000 children aged 6 to 14 years in one area of Italy and found that only one half of the 38 children with epilepsy had a normal scholastic record. One third of the children were in special classes, nearly all because of mental handicap. Stores and Hart (1976) did not find any deterioration of reading skills in a group of children with generalized epilepsy compared with matched controls, but children with focal spikes had impaired reading accuracy. Seidenberg et al. (1986) found that 122 children with epilepsy were, as a group, making less academic progress than expected for their age and IQ. Their greatest difficulties were in arithmetic, followed by spelling, reading, comprehension and word recognition. Corbett et al. (1975) found that the prevalence of epilepsy depended on the degree of mental handicap. Nineteen per cent of those with IQ less than 50 had seizures in the preceding year. For IQ 35 to 50 the figure was 15%, IQ 20 to 35 it was 26% and for those with IQ less than 20, seizures were recorded in the preceding year in 27%. This study appears to show a clear association between degree of mental handicap and prevalence of seizures in children. The association between seizures and intellectual deterioration has been studied by Corbett and co-workers (1985, 1986). Despite the fact that some of these studies used highly selected samples of children, an association between cognitive impairment and epilepsy in at least some groups of children seems indisputable. Such an association does not, however, answer the questions regarding causality.

DOES EPILEPSY CAUSE DETERIORATION?

In a recent review assessing aspects of dementia in adults, Mclean (1987) lists the causes of dementia from pooled data on 1306 patients. Epilepsy is stated as the identified cause in five cases. In contrast Ellenberg et al. (1985), from data collected in the National Collaborative Perinatal Project, appeared to reach the conclusion that seizures do not cause intellectual deterioration in children. This again raises the question of whether the studies in which epilepsy and intellectual deterioration were associated selected their patients in such a way that both epilepsy and intellectual impairment were present with no causal relationship between them. The most likely explanation is that a sub-group of children with epilepsy did deteriorate because of the epilepsy although this point is difficult to prove. In a prospective study, Bourgeois et al. (1983) tested 72 children within two weeks of the diagnosis of epilepsy and at yearly intervals thereafter, for an average of four years. They found that the initial IQ was not significantly different from that of siblings but eight patients (11%) had a fall in IQ of 10 points or more. These children differed significantly from the others in having an earlier age of seizure onset and a higher incidence of drug levels in the toxic range.

DOES DETERIORATION CAUSE EPILEPSY?

This question may, at first sight, appear to be a trivial one. It is quite obvious, for example that trauma can cause brain damage and that the brain damage in turn can result in epilepsy. Similarly central nervous system infections, such as meningitis, can cause brain damage and epilepsy. In adults, the all too common condition of Alzheimer's disease frequently results in seizures. The devastating condition of subacute sclerosing panencephalitis also results in progressive neurological deterioration with accompaning seizures. Corbett (1985) has listed some other specific conditions in which obvious brain abnormality is almost certainly responsible for the epilepsy. In childhood, diseases of the grey matter, e.g. Batten's disease, are an important, although uncommon cause of brain deterioration and epilepsy. The difficulty arises when considering a small group of children who deteriorate for no apparent cause and who have seizures. Some of these children have not been treated with anticonvulsants prior to the deterioration and consequently medication cannot be responsible. They have not had bouts of status epilepticus, nor is there any evidence of 'sub-clinical' status and they do not have any recognizable metabolic, infective, chromosomal or structural cause for the deterioration or the epilepsy. Gordon and the present author (unpublished) have identified some patients in whom this abnormal pattern is found to be associated by a partial aryl sulphatase A deficiency which is both biochemically and clinically quite different from metachromatic leucodystrophy. This is not one of the recognized neurodegen-erative conditions described in the textbooks. If clinicians continue to discover more and more previously unknown neurodegenerative disorders these might account for an increasing proportion of children with epilepsy who undergo cognitive deterioration.

WHEN EPILEPSY AND COGNITIVE IMPAIRMENT OCCUR TOGETHER WHICH FACTORS MIGHT BE IMPORTANT?

Preceding organic brain damage

Lennox (1942) compared 449 'symptomatic' epilepsy patients with 1456 'essential' epilepsy patients. He found 26% of the symptomatic group and 10% of the essential group showed definite deterioration. Lennox and Collins (1945) compared the IQ of twins with and without epilepsy. They found that the average IQ if neither twin had epilepsy was 109. If one had epilepsy and the other did not the respective average IQ scores were 103 and 96. For those with epilepsy and brain damage the average IQ was 77. This study, whilst certainly interesting in its own right, does not answer many questions regarding the association between seizures and cognitive impairment since it would be expected that the twin who suffered greater birth trauma would be subject both to greater brain damage and a higher chance of epilepsy.

Yacorzynski and Arieff (1942) carried out sequential IQ tests on adults with 'organic' and non-organic epilepsy. The organic group were defined as showing neurological signs of brain damage. Thirty-seven per cent of the organic group deteriorated compared with 6% of the non-organic group. Although the IQ fall associated with the deteriorating group was small, viz. 6 points, this study is interesting in its confirmation of the suggestion that the already damaged brain might be more susceptible to further damage by seizures (see introduction). Collins (1951) studied 400 patients with epilepsy and concluded that there was little evidence of deterioration except in the organic cases. Chaudhry and Pond (1961) stated that there is a tendency for the already dull child to deteriorate more than the child who is average or above. Matsumoto et al. (1983), in their study of the prognosis of seizures commencing in the first year of life, emphasized that the outcome of secondary generalized epilepsy was poor. This finding was confirmed by O'Leary et al. (1983) amongst others.

Age of seizure onset

Lennox (1942) showed that the earlier the seizure onset in patients with either symptomatic or idiopathic epilepsy, the greater the proportion who deteriorated. Collins (1951) found a positive correlation of IQ with age of seizure onset and a very low negative correlation with the duration of the seizures.

Keith et al. (1955) collected data on 296 children attending the Mayo Clinic and found a strong relationship between the age of seizure onset and intellectual impairment. Sixty-five per cent of those with onset under 6 months had intellectual impairment compared with 49% for onset 6 months to 2 years, 34%

for onset 2–4 years, 22% for onset 4–7 years and 12% for onset between 7–15 years. The age groupings in this study are open to question since the first two groups would both overlap with the age range in which hypsarrhythmia is likely to occur with its high probability of mental handicap. The figures are nevertheless interesting. These authors make the point that the proportion with mental handicap was much higher in the symptomatic group (73%) than in the idiopathic group (22.2%).

Rodin (1968) also found that greater intellectual impairment was associated with earlier seizure onset, correcting for duration of seizures. Hung (1968) carried out a detailed clinic-based study on 500 Chinese patients and concluded that early seizure onset, not the duration of the seizure disorder, was associated with a high incidence of intellectual impairment. This was true both for mild and severe impairment. Dikmen et al. (1975) found that early seizure onset, 0–5 years, was associated with poorer scores on cognitive testing in adulthood than later onset (17–50 years). This study, unlike that of Hung (1968), does not separate age of onset from duration of seizure disorder. Harrison and Taylor (1976) emphasized that early childhood seizures could have a poor long-term prognosis on several different criteria, including intellectual outcome. In a follow-up report, Chevrie and Aicardi (1972) reported a poor prognosis for seizures commencing in the first year of life even if infantile spasms were excluded. This was confirmed by Matsumoto et al. (1983).

O'Leary et al. (1983) examined 106 children, comparing verbal and performance IQs for early and late onset seizures. There was no difference between the verbal IQ for early and late onset partial seizures but the performance IQ was less for early onset. For generalized seizures both the VIQ and PIQ were lower for the early onset group.

The population based study of Ellenberg et al. (1985) showed no significant effect of age of seizure onset on cognitive function. In a prospective study, Bourgeois et al. (1983) found that the eight children who deteriorated by more than 10 points in IQ had earlier seizure onset as one of the best predictors.

Duration of epilepsy

Various authors have used different criteria related to the duration of epilepsy. Age of onset, duration of seizure disorder, number of years with seizures and total number of seizures are all interrelated variables. Some studies have examined these variables separately and others have not. Dikmen and Matthews (1977) applied a number of cognitive tests to 72 patients with major motor seizures. The high-risk group for severe generalized cognitive impairment had a long seizure history, early age of onset and high seizure frequency or any combination of two of these factors. Hung (1968) evaluated age of seizure onset and duration of epilepsy separately and concluded that the former was a significant factor associated with intellectual impairment but the latter was not.

Farwell et al. (1985) assessed 118 children aged 6 to 15 years. More of the variance in IQ fall was associated with duration of seizure disorder than with age of onset.

Seizure type

Children with the West syndrome of hypsarrhythmia/infantile spasms have a poor prognosis for subsequent intellectual development. Approximately 90% will have significant intellectual impairment. Illingworth (1955) has described in detail several of these children with seizure onset between 4 and 8 months. He emphasized that both intellectual deterioration and seizures can begin with little or no warning and that many of these children appeared totally normal beforehand. It would appear that, in these cases, the seizures do not cause the intellectual deterioration nor does the intellectual deterioration cause the seizures, but there is some quite rapidly occurring underlying process causing both. An excellent and detailed review of infantile spasms has been carried out by Jeavons and Bower (1964). A significant proportion of children with the West syndrome are not neurologically normal before the onset of the seizures and Matsumoto et al. (1981) have pointed out that these children have a worse prognosis for subsequent cognitive development.

The Lennox–Gastaut syndrome (Lennox, 1945; Gibbs and Gibbs, 1962; Gastaut et al., 1966) has a typical age of onset between 2 and 6 years with minor motor seizures consisting of absences, myoclonic jerks and akinetic seizures. The EEG shows low frequency spike and wave complexes at 1.5–2.5 Hz and the condition is resistant to anticonvulsants with 80–90% of the children becoming intellectually impaired. In 20–30% it is preceded by infantile spasms. Although Chevrie and Aicardi (1972) have pointed out that this is not a homogeneous entity, it is clear that a high proportion of children who have the syndrome undergo serious cognitive deterioration. It can again be argued that this might reflect some underlying unidentified degenerative brain process although in many cases there is no evidence for this suggestion. In other cases the condition is clearly secondary to some brain insult. Whether the excessive metabolic demands of the frequent abnormal electrical discharges seen in this syndrome can cause the deterioration is a matter for debate.

Matthews and Kløve (1976) found that patients with major motor seizures of unknown aetiology performed more poorly on cognitive testing than did normal controls but patients with psychomotor seizures of unknown aetiology produced results comparable to those of normal controls. Collins (1951) found that, although IQ differences were small, subjects with petit mal epilepsy scored the highest with those who had psychomotor epilepsy being intermediate and those with major seizures scoring a little lower. O'Leary et al. (1983) compared cognitive tests on children with generalized and partial seizures. They found that early onset generalized seizures were associated with lower IQ results than early onset partial seizures. Giordani et al. (1985) tested 350 subjects aged 9 to 40 on the WISC and WAIS. They examined performance on the various sub-tests in relationship to seizure type and found that children with primary generalized seizures and secondarily generalized seizures performed worse on digit span, arithmetic, block design, object assembly and coding than those with partial seizures. Farwell et al. (1985) tested 118 children and found that lower IQ was associated with atypical absences, myoclonic seizures and drop attacks in contrast to generalized tonic-clonic seizures, typical absences and partial seizures or combinations of these, which were associated with near average IQ.

Seizure frequency

Dodrill and Troupin (1976), in twin studies, found that the twin with more frequent seizures performed worse on tests of cognitive function. As previously discussed, this might reflect greater underlying brain damage causing the seizures rather than indicating causality in the opposite direction. Chaudhry and Pond (1961) comparing 28 children who had epilepsy and deterioration with a control group who did not deteriorate concluded that increased seizure frequency was statistically related to the deterioration. In examining the failure of children with epilepsy to reach their expected academic achievement, Seidenberg et al. (1986) found that lifetime total seizure frequency was a strong correlate. Farwell et al. (1985) in a clinic based study on 118 children with epilepsy aged 6 to 15 years found a highly significant inverse correlation between years with seizures and intelligence. Hung (1968) found a highly significant relationship between the incidence of mental impairment and seizure frequency.

Anti-epileptic drug effects

Anti-epileptic drug effects on cognitive deterioration can be divided into acute reversible effects and chronic effects. Stores (1971) found that phenytoin appeared to be associated with adverse effects on intellectual processes. Stores and Hart (1976) confirmed an association between lower reading skills and this drug. Corbett et al. (1985), in a study of cognitive deterioration in 312 children at Lingfield Hospital School, found an association between long-term pheny-toin therapy and cognitive deterioration.

It is difficult to compensate entirely for confounding factors when examining both the epilepsy and the chronic effects of anticonvulsant drugs since people with more severe brain damage and more difficult to control seizures are likely to be treated with polypharmacy in higher dosage. Some of these difficulties can be overcome by using healthy volunteers, as in the studies by Thompson (1981) but this assesses acute effects. Nonetheless, these confirmed the adverse effect of phenytoin on cognitive function. In patients on monotherapy, Thompson and Trimble (1982) compared the effects of carbamazepine, sodium valproate and phenytoin on tests of cognitive function. At high serum levels of phenytoin and sodium valproate performance deteriorated. Carbamazepine did not seem to be associated with such deterioration. Bourgeois et al. (1983) (see earlier) reported a high incidence of drug levels in the toxic range as being one of the best predictors of deterioration in IQ. Andrewes et al. (1986) found that subjects taking phenytoin performed less well on memory tests than those taking carbamazepine.

Head injury in seizures

In the sub-group of children with epilepsy and intellectual deterioration, a number certainly have experienced repeated head injury through falling in seizures. Atonic drop attacks are of particular concern but head injury may also occur in tonic seizures when the head may fall in a long arc to the ground. Head injury can occur in other types of seizures, e.g. simple motor seizures of the lower limb causing a fall. It is difficult to quantify the effect of head injury on the brain. A fall which causes soft tissue injury and copious bleeding might cause less brain trauma than an apparently trivial injury in a person whose brain is shrunken and poorly cushioned by the skull. Attempts to obtain some quantitative measure of brain damage by assaying the blood level of brain enzymes might be helpful in this regard (Forsyth, private communication). Whilst there is no doubt that repeated head trauma can cause permanent brain damage, as is clearly demonstrated by some boxers, the relative importance of this factor in causing cognitive deterioration in children with epilepsy has still to be evaluated.

STATE-DEPENDENT OR VARIABLE COGNITIVE IMPAIRMENT IN CHILDREN

Both epilepsy related phenomena and anti-epileptic medication can cause variable cognitive impairment. Drugs such as phenobarbitone, primidone and the benzodiazepines can affect awareness and concentration, in turn affecting cognitive performance. Even drugs which are not usually sedative can do so if the blood levels reach the toxic range. These acute, reversible effects of anti-epileptic drugs are well discussed elsewhere, notably in a series of papers by Trimble, Thompson and their co-workers and in a recent paper by Rodin et al. (1986). Tylor Fox (1924) commented on the variability of performance of children with epilepsy. Apart from the more obvious ictal and post-ictal states, in which awareness is quite clearly impaired, some individuals may be subject to any of a variety of changes in mood or awareness related to their seizures. During the prodrome, which typically lasts between hours and a day or two, the individual may become very irritable with a poor concentration span. Good studies on the effect of the prodrome on cognition are difficult to perform, since the state is rather non-specific and cannot be predicted in time.

The work of Stores and Hart (1976) has already been discussed. They found an association between left-sided spikes and reading ability. It is quite plausible to extend this argument by suggesting that, on occasions when frequent abnormal discharges are present in any part of the brain, cognitive function subserved by that area might be temporarily impaired. Binnie and co-workers (see Chapter 4) have carried out some fascinating work on transitory cognitive impairment, showing that brief epileptiform discharges can effect performance on verbal or non-verbal tasks, depending on the location of the discharges. The phenomenon of non-convulsive status, either complex partial seizure status or absence status, is now becoming more widely recognized. Although some children who enter this state show little outward sign of it, others can become quite 'zombie-like' with seriously impaired abilities whilst it continues.

After major seizures, a brief period of confusion is common. However, some children have quite prolonged periods in which they may wander around in a trance-like state, clinically consistent with the definition of a fugue state, containing the elements of wandering, impaired awareness and subsequent amnesia for events during the episode. These postictal fugue states may last several days, particularly after a cluster of seizures, and are not responsive to medication once they are established. They can sometimes be prevented by preventing clusters of seizures, for example giving diazepam or clobazam after the first seizure or two, stopping subsequent seizures in the cluster. Postictal and interictal schizophreniform psychoses and affective states can also affect performance on cognitive tests in a major and variable way.

ONGOING STUDIES OF COGNITIVE DETERIORATION IN CHILDREN WITH EPILEPSY AT LINGFIELD HOSPITAL SCHOOL

The classical studies of Tylor Fox have already been discussed in an earlier section. Corbett et al. (1985b) carried out a further study together with the current author and others on the children at Lingfield Hospital. This was in part a follow-up to an earlier study carried out in 1976 (Corbett et al., 1985a). The total number of children with epilepsy was 201, the age range 5 to 19 and the mean age 13. Thirty-nine per cent had IQ scores less than 50, 39% were in the range 50–70 and 22% had IQs above 70. Sequential IQ results were available for 160 in this study, of whom 80 (50%) deteriorated by more than 15 points and 25 (16%) deteriorated by more than 30 points.

Examination of the following factors revealed no significant relationship to IQ: age, sex, initial IQ, age of seizure onset, seizure frequency, EEG abnormality and anticonvulsants. It should be noted, in contrast to the 1976 cohort

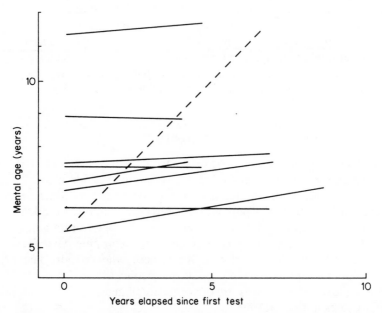

Fig. 1   Mental age plotted against years since initial test on WISC-R. The expected slope is shown by the interrupted line at 45°.

(Corbett et al., 1985a) that no relationship was found between chronic pheny-toin administration and cognitive deterioration. However, the use of phenytoin had declined markedly in the intervening years and the lack of a statistically significant relationship may reflect the smaller number of children who were taking this drug in the later study.

In an ongoing study by the current author and co-workers, sequential raw scores for some of these children have been compared over a period of time ranging from 3 to 8 years. A close examination of eight students who had apparently deteriorated and for whom sequential raw score data were avail-able, reveals that the children seem almost to have undergone intellectual arrest. This is shown clearly in Figure 1 which plots the mental age against time elapsed since the first assessment. The expected slope of the lines is 45°, but they are almost horizontal. Because the mental age hardly increases at all, the IQ appears progressively to fall. The concept of developmental arrest in children goes very much against the grain of paediatric thinking which tends to compare development by referring to centile lines, and to define deterioration as being a downward departure from the centiles. Developmental arrest would properly be considered as deterioration using these criteria, although skills are not necessarily lost. The group for which full data are available is small. It remains to be seen whether the concept of developmental arrest will apply to a larger number of the sub-group of children who show progressive IQ fall. Some of the children in the Lingfield study have clearly deteriorated as a result of status epilepticus occurring before they arrived in an establishment where prompt treatment was unavailable. In one such case the epilepsy followed a road traffic accident but intellect was normal before the subject experienced a prolonged seizure, lasting 45 minutes, after which it had clearly deteriorated. The importance of prompt treatment of status epilepticus in childhood cannot be overemphasized.

CONCLUSIONS

Although useful conclusions can be drawn from the large amount of literature published on the subject of cognitive deterioration in children with epilepsy, there is a need for further systematic prospective studies in which sequential data are collected. Ideally, a population-based group should be used to identify the small sub-group of children with epilepsy who deteriorate and this sub-group should be examined in greater detail to determine what factors differentiate children who deteriorate from those who do not. The present situation can be summarized in the following conclusions:

1. Most children with epilepsy are of normal intelligence and their intellectual ability does not deteriorate.
2. Because of this, group epidemiological studies are unlikely to demonstrate any effect of epilepsy on intellectual functioning.
3. A small sub-group of children who have epilepsy do deteriorate intellectually.
4. Some of the children with epilepsy who deteriorate have recognized pre-existing brain damage but some do not.
5. Absence seizures, unaccompanied by seizures of other types, probably have a good prognosis. Infantile spasms and the Lennox–Gastaut syndrome generally have a poor prognosis for future intellect. Mixed epilepsy, when several seizure types occur together also probably has a poor prognosis.
6. Status epilepticus can undoubtedly cause intellectual and neurological deterioration.
7. There is a possibility that phenytoin causes a chronic encephalopathy with intellectual deterioration.
8. Whenever a child deteriorates intellectually, with or without seizures, the possibility of cerebral pathology must always be considered, e.g. neurodegenerative disease, brain tumour.
9. In those children with epilepsy who do deteriorate, although there is conflicting evidence, the literature suggests that early age of onset, frequent seizures, prolonged seizures, association with pre-existing brain damage and mixed seizure type may all contribute to the intellectual deterioration.

REFERENCES

ADDY, D. (1987) Cognitive function in children with epilepsy. *Dev. Med. Child Neurol.*, **29**, 394–404.

ANDREWES, D.G., BULLEN, J.G., TOMLINSON, L., ELWES, R.D. and REYNOLDS, E.H. (1986) A comparative study of the cognitive effects of phenytoin and carbamazepine in new referrals with epilepsy. *Epilepsia*, **27**, 128–134.

BOURGEOIS, B.F.D., PRENSKY, A.L., PALKES, H.S., TALENT, B.K. and BUSCH, S.G. (1983) Intelligence in epilepsy: a prospective study in children. *Ann. Neurol.*, **14**, 438–444.

BROWN, S.W. and REYNOLDS, E.H. (1981) Cognitive impairment in epileptic patients. In *Epilepsy and Psychiatry* (eds E.H. REYNOLDS and M. TRIMBLE), Churchill-Livingstone, Edinburgh.

CHAUDHRY, M.R. and POND, D.A. (1961) Mental deterioration in epileptic children. *J. Neurol. Neurosurg. Psychiat.*, **24**, 213–219.

CHEVRIE, J.J. and AIRCARDI, J. (1972) Childhood epileptic encephalopathy with slow spike-wave. A statistical study of 80 cases. *Epilepsia*, **13**, 259–271.

COLLINS, A.L. (1951) Epileptic intelligence, *J. Consult. Psychol.*, **15**, 392–399.

COOKSON, S.H. (1927) An analysis of 100 cases of fits in children. *Arch. Dis. Child.*, **II**, 178.

CORBETT, J.A. (1985) Epilepsy as part of a handicapping condition. In *Paediatric Perspectives on Epilepsy* (eds E. ROSS and E. REYNOLDS), John Wiley and Sons, Chichester.

CORBETT, J.A., HARRIS, R. and ROBINSON, R. (1975) Epilepsy. In *Mental Retardation and Developmental Disabilities*, **VII**, 79–111 (ed. J. WORTIS). Bruner Mazel, New York.

CORBETT, J.A., TRIMBLE, M.R., and NICHOL, T.C. (1985a) Behavioural and cognitive impairments in children with epilepsy: The long-term effects of anticonvulsant therapy. *J. Am. Acad. Child. Psychiat.*, **24**, 17–23.

CORBETT, J.A., BESAG, F.M.C., JAMES, A. and WHITE, S. (1985b) Cognitive and behavioural impairment in children with epilepsy. Lingfield study II – Preliminary analysis. Paper presented at British Paediatric Neurology Association, January.

CORBETT, J.A., BESAG, F.M.C., FOWLER, M., GOODMAN, R. and JAMES, A. (1986) Dementia in Epilepsy? Paper presented at Northern European Epilepsy Conference, York.

DAWSON, S. and CONN, J.C.M. (1929) The intelligence of epileptic children. *Arch. Dis. Child.*, **4**, 142–151.

DIKMEN, S. and MATTHEWS, C.G. (1977) Effect of major motor seizure frequency upon cognitive-intellectual functions in adults. *Epilepsia*, **18**, 21–29.

DIKMEN, S., MATTHEWS, C.G. and HARLEY, J.P. (1975) The effect of early versus late onset of major motor epilepsy upon cognitive-intellectual performance. *Epilepsia*, **16**, 73–81.

DODRILL, C.B. and TROUPIN, A.S. (1976) Seizures and adaptive abilities, *Arch. Neurol.*, **33**, 604–607.

ELLENBERG, J.H., HIRTZ, D.G. and NELSON, K.B. (1985) Do seizures in children cause intellectual deterioration? *Ann. Neurol.*, **18**, 389.

FARWELL, J.R., DODRILL, C.B. and BATZEL, L.W. (1985) Neuropsychological abilities of children with epilepsy. *Epilepsia*, **26**, 395–400.

GASTAUT, H., ROGER, J., SOULAYROL, R., TASSINARI, C.A., REGIS, H., DRAVET, C., BERNARD, R., PINSARD, N. and SAINT-JEAN, M. (1966) Childhood epileptic encephalopathy with diffuse spike-waves (otherwise known as 'petit mal variant') or Lennox syndrome. *Epilepsia*, **7**, 139–179.

GIBBS, F.A. and GIBBS, E.L. (1962) *Atlas of Electroencephalography*. 2. Addison-Wesley, Reading, Massachusetts.

GIORDANI, B., BERENT, S., SACKELLARES, J.C., ROURKE, D., SEIDENBERG, M., O'LEARY, D.S., DREIFUSS, F.E. and BOLL, T.J. (1985) Intelligence test performance of patients with partial and generalized seizures. *Epilepsia*, **26**, 37–42.

HARRISON, R.M. and TAYLOR, D.C. (1976) Childhood seizures: a 25-year follow-up, *Lancet*, **ii**, 948–951.

HUNG, T.-P. (1968) Intellectual impairment and behaviour disorder in 500 epileptic patients. *Proc. Aust. Assoc. Neurol.*, **5**, 163–170.

ILLINGWORTH, R.S. (1955) Sudden mental deterioration with convulsions in infancy. *Arch. Dis. Child.*, **30**, 529–537.

JEAVONS, P.M. and BOWER, B.D. (1964) *Infantile Spasms. Clinics in Developmental Medicine.* No. 15, Spastics Soc. Med. Ed. Info. Unit with Heinemann Medical, London.

KEITH, H.M., EWERT, J.C., GREEN, M.W. and GAGE, R.P. (1955) Mental status of children with convulsive disorders. *Neurology (Minneapolis)*, **5**, 419–425.

LENNOX, W.G. (1942) Brain injury drugs and environment as causes of mental decay in epileptics. *Am. J. Psychiat.*, **99**, 174–180.

LENNOX, W.G. and COLLINS, A.L. (1945) Intelligence of normal and epileptic twins. *Am. J. Psychiat.*, **10**, 764–769.

LESSER, R.P., LUDERS, H., WYLLIE, E., DINNER, D.S. and MORRIS III, H.H. (1986) Mental deterioration in epilepsy. *Epilepsia*, **27**, (suppl. 2), S105–S123.

McLEAN, S. (1987) Review: Assessing dementia. Part 1: Difficulties, definitions and differential diagnosis. *Aust. N.Z. J. Psychiat.*, **21**, 142–174.

MATSUMOTO, A., WATANABE, K., NEGORO, T., SUGIURA, M., IWASE, K., HARA, K. and MIYAZAKI, S. (1981) Long-term prognosis after infantile spasms: A statistical study of prognostic factors in 200 cases. *Dev. Med. Child. Neurol.*, **23**, 51–65.

MATSUMOTO, A., WATANABE, K., SUGIURA, M., NEGORO, T., TAKAESU, E. and IWASE, K. (1983) Long-term prognosis of convulsive disorders in the first year of life: Mental and physical development and seizure persistence. *Epilepsia*, **24**, 321–329.

MATTHEWS, C.G. and KLØVE, H. (1967) Differential psychological performances in major motor, psychomotor, and mixed seizure classification of known and unknown etiology. *Epilepsia*, **8**, 117–128.

O'LEARY, D.S., LOVELL, M.R., SACKELLARES, J.C., BERENT, S., GIORDANI, B., SEIDENBERG, M. and BOLL, T.J. (1983) Effects of age of onset of partial and generalized seizures on neuropsychological performance in children. *J. Nerv. Ment. Dis.*, **171**, 624–629.

PAZZAGLIA, P. and FRANK-PAZZAGLIA, L. (1976) Record in grade school of pupils with epilepsy: An epidemiological study. *Epilepsia*, **17**, 361–366.

POND, D.A. and BIDWELL, B.H. (1959/60) A survey of epilepsy in fourteen general practices. II. Social and psychological aspects. *Epilepsia*, **1**, 285–299.

RODIN, E.A. (1968) *The Prognosis of Patients with Epilepsy.* C. Thomas, Springfield, Illinois.

RODIN, E.A., SCHMALTZ, S. and TWITTY, G. (1986) Intellectual functions of patients with childhood-onset epilepsy. *Dev. Med. Child. Neurol.*, **28**, 25–33.

RUTTER, M., GRAHAM, P. and YULE, W. (1970) A neuropsychiatric study in childhood. *Clinics in Developmental Medicine*, Nos 35/36 SIMP with Heinemann Medical, London.

SEIDENBERG, M., BECK, N., GEISSER, M., GIORDANI, B., SACKELLARES, J.C., BERENT, S., DREIFUSS, F.E. and BOLL, T.J. (1986) Academic achievement of children with epilepsy. *Epilepsia*, **27**, 753–759.

STORES, G. (1971) Cognitive function in children with epilepsy. *Dev. Med. Child. Neurol.*, **13**, 390–393.

STORES, G. and HART, J. (1976) Reading skills of children with generalised or focal epilepsy attending ordinary school. *Dev. Med. Child. Neurol.*, **18**, 705–716.

THOMPSON, P.J. (1981) The effects of anticonvulsant drugs on the cognitive functioning of normal volunteers and patients with epilepsy. PhD Thesis, University of London.

THOMPSON, P.J. and TRIMBLE, M.R. (1982) Comparative effects of anticonvulsant drugs on cognitive testing. *Br. J. Clin. Pract.*, Suppl. **18**, 154–156.

TYLOR FOX, J. (1924) The response of epileptic children to mental and educational tests. *Br. J. Med. Psychol.*, **4**, 235–238.

YACORZYNSKI, G.K. and ARIEFF, A.J. (1942) Absence of deterioration in patients with non-organic epilepsy with especial reference to bromide therapy. *J. Nerv. Ment. Dis.*, **95**, 687–697.

Discussion

Section III

Ms J. Ossetin: Dr Besag, could you clarify the difference between the concept of mental arrest and intellectual deterioration. Your graph actually shows that these children do develop, albeit at a much slower rate than ordinary children, for whatever reason.

Dr F.M.C. Besag: First of all, plotting the IQ would clearly show a fall, because the mental age is remaining more or less stationary, but chronological age is increasing with the young subjects. So, by usual standards these people are deteriorating because their IQ is falling. If you look at the raw scores, however, their mental age is more or less stationary. That was the reason for saying that these children arrested. I agree some of them creep up a little bit, but the slope of the curve was so low that this is intellectual arrest. It is something that Professor Corbett recognized many years ago, but there is an ongoing argument about this.

Dr I. McKinlay (Manchester): I am interested in Dr Ross's figures about the proportions of children with epilepsy going to special schools. In Salford, where I have been making a study, there are just over 200 children with epilepsy, and 98 are in special schools, 60 of them in schools for children with severe learning difficulties. The others who are in special schools are not only placed there because of epilepsy, but for other reasons, either learning difficulties or attachment disorders or whatever. The other thing that I found interesting looking at the whole population with epilepsy in special schools is that the proportion in schools for children with moderate learning difficulties, in the Greater Manchester area, is 5½ per cent, which compares with 18 per cent in Sweden. It seems in Sweden, that the social disadvantage element which leads many people in this country to go into special schools is less prominent and we have a greater dilution of people with brain disorders in our special schools for social reasons than is the case in other countries.

Dr F.M.C. Besag: The students coming to Lingfield have changed very markedly, even over a ten-year period. We get many more disabled children for reasons other than epilepsy.

Dr E.M. Ross: I think part of the difficulty is getting the denominator of the equation because many children with epilepsy are unknown to schools. In a hospital series I looked at we found only a fraction of what I would have expected from national study figures. A lot of parents are very against their child's epilepsy being declared to the school. I do my utmost to encourage parents to share this information with the school, but it is not something that one can force upon them. I think you are bound to have 'secret' people with epilepsy in Salford, and it makes the collecting of data difficult. To what extent we gathered all the people with epilepsy must be open to question. When we wrote to people at age 28 with epilepsy and said: 'We would like to come and see you again and, in a very roundabout way, have you ever had a fit etc. again?' – a lot of them said 'No, I've never had one in my life', and yet we have clearcut evidence that when they were younger, they had a seizure disorder.

Dr D.B. Smith: Dr Besag, you mentioned that status epilepticus was associated with intellectual deterioration. Did you differentiate between tonic-clonic status epilepticus and a so-called ictal confusional state, or non-motor status epilepticus?

Dr F.M.C. Besag: I find it very worrying if we see a lot of epileptic activity on the EEG over very long periods of time. I think probably the latter do deteriorate.

Dr S.H. Green (Birmingham): Dr Besag, what do you think we can learn from certain special models, like tuberous sclerosis where there is quite a clear association between epilepsy and retardation; it appears that one does not get retardation without the epilepsy?

Dr F.M.C. Besag: That would be a very interesting model to study.

Dr D. Mellor (Nottingham): A word of caution. The difficulty would be that it is the child who has epilepsy and tuberous sclerosis who has the more severe tuberous sclerosis in a condition which has a very wide range of expression. Therefore we would be looking perhaps not at the effect of epilepsy but at the effect of severe tuberous sclerosis.

Dr S.H. Green: A classic paper from the Mayo Clinic, looking at twins with tuberous sclerosis and epilepsy, suggested that having the epilepsy accounted for the deterioration in the twin.

Dr F.M.C. Besag: Again it is sequential data that one needs.

Dr D. Mellor: But even with sequential data there is a problem. We know that tuberous sclerosis is a progressive condition, with the appearance of tumours on the CT scans with the passage of time.

Dr M.R. Trimble: Dr Besag, you have discussed patients with an abnormal mental state which goes on sometimes for days or longer. Is this epilepsy, and are they having seizures? I suggest that the pathology or the underlying pathophysiology and neuro-chemistry of these states are entirely different from that which produces 'the seizure' which is the hallmark of clinical epilepsy.

Dr F.M.C. Besag: That is a fascinating question, to which we do not have the answer. What is a 'brief paroxysmal event' in the definition of a seizure. These are paroxysmal, but can last for a fortnight.

Dr S. Wallis (Reading): No one has mentioned the recent neurochemical investigations of Meldrum and others, which have shown that you can have neurotoxic amino acids, which are present with a spike discharge. This may be related to the possible intellectual and neurological arrests or deterioration which occur in children with epilepsy.

Dr M.R. Trimble: I would like to comment further on the question of intellectual deterioration or arrest. Aside from epilepsy there are a number of other conditions in neuropsychiatry where one sees the same phenomenon. Schizophrenia is an excellent example. People can deteriorate in adolescence, but they reach a stage where they are burnt out. Their intellectual decline does not progress any further. I think the pathology of these states is entirely different from the pathology of senile dementia or other progressive neurological conditions.

Professor J.A. Corbett: I think they are what we called 'non-progressive disintegrative disorder'. Rather than using the term 'dementia infantalis'; the term dementia should be restricted to conditions occurring in adult life. Dr Green has views about these interruptions in development, some of which progress. We have a group of children who most clearly illustrated this by their reading age. They suddenly stick at a reading age of six; they attain that vocabulary and they never learn anything more.

Dr S.H. Green: It is a very difficult area. I am often asked by school teachers about children who have been seen by a psychologist who says that their IQ has dropped, and the parents have said the same. Another way of looking at it is that these children might have achieved their final level rather earlier than others, and they have a lower 'ceiling' than other children, but they are not deteriorating in the same way as a child with progressive dementia. I think there are different categories. What the neurochemistry of this is, I do not know. But it is interesting that there are a few neurometabolic diseases which can actually burn out. I remember seeing two children at an end-stage plateau. It turned out that they had a variety of Batten's Disease.

Professor N. O'Donohoe (Dublin): Some children arrest when they have epilepsy with encephalitis. I have certainly seen this.

Section IV

10

Anticonvulsant drugs: mood and cognitive function

MICHAEL R. TRIMBLE
National Hospitals for Nervous Diseases and Institute of Neurology, London

INTRODUCTION

In recent years the fact that patients with epilepsy may suffer from cognitive disruption or behaviour disturbances has become accepted. Although there is much speculation as to the role of various factors in relationship to these problems, little systematic research has been carried out. With regards to cognitive function, even the influence of some basic variables such as seizure site and seizure frequency have yet to be clarified, and with regards to behaviour, the persistent debates over the role of temporal lobe disturbances in provoking changes of personality or psychosis continue (Trimble, 1985).

Although anticonvulsant drugs have always been suspected as being of relevance with regards to cognitive and behaviour changes, it is only in recent years that their influence has become an area of active research interest (Trimble and Reynolds, 1976). It is intended here to review some of the recent literature and attempt to come to some conclusions with regards to the current state of knowledge regarding the role of anticonvulsant drugs on these variables.

COGNITIVE FUNCTION

Studies with individual drugs

Several groups have evolved different strategies to investigate the influence of anticonvulsant drugs on cognitive function. In a series of studies carried out at the National Hospitals, we have investigated volunteers and patients receiving monotherapy using a psychological test battery specifically constructed for examining changes in neuropsychological function using a longitudinal design (Thompson and Trimble, 1982a, b; Thompson and Trimble, 1983). In one investigation, patients were seen on two occasions at an interval separated by three months. Patients were given psychological testing on a battery which included memory, attention and concentration, perceptual speed, decision-making speed and motor speed tasks. Following the testing patients had their drug regime changed, approximately half increasing the dose of drug received, the other half decreasing it. Thus, all patients were seen on two occasions, once at a high and once at a low serum level. The patients were on monotherapy with either phenytoin, sodium valproate or carbamazepine, and differences in performance between the high and low serum level session were evaluated. The level at the high serum level session was approximately twice that of the low serum level one. Deficits in performance were observed in association with the high serum level session, most marked for patients on phenytoin and sodium valproate, even though the mean serum levels of these drugs were within the therapeutic ranges at both testing sessions. In contrast, carbamazepine-treated patients showed minimal changes of performance between high and low serum level sessions, and in some of the tasks, in which significant impairments were noted with phenytoin or sodium valproate, the trend was for higher levels of carbamazepine to be associated with improved performance. Impairment at high levels on this drug were recorded for two measures, one reflecting manual speed, the other being the Stroop test.

In studies using volunteers, using the same or a modified psychological test battery, subjects were given anticonvulsant drugs and matching placebo tablets for a period of two weeks in a double-blind crossover design. Psychological testing took place before and on completion of the treatment phases, and at the end of the testing sessions serum levels were assessed in order to check compliance. In these investigations, from a homogeneous subject pool, we have examined phenytoin, carbamazepine, sodium valproate, clonazepam and clobazam (Thompson et al., 1981; Thompson and Trimble, 1981; Cull and Trimble, 1985; Cull and Trimble, 1988). Some significant deficits of performance were recorded for all drugs, but impairments were most marked following phenytoin and clonazepam. For phenytoin, impairments occurred on measures of memory, mental and motor speed at a dose of 100 mg three times a day. These changes were observed at a mean anticonvulsant level just below the quoted therapeutic range. Using a modified psychological test battery, employing microcomputers for the delivery of test stimuli, clonazepam (0.5 mgms tds) was shown to impair mental speed, central cognitive processing ability, memory and perceptuomotor performance. Again, with both drugs, significant correlations were noted between serum levels and the degree of deterioration on test performance on some of the measures. With sodium valproate and carbamazepine, significant impairments in test performance occurred on four and two measures respectively, with mean anticonvulsant levels within the therapeutic ranges. For clobazam, less in the way of changes were seen, and in contrast to clonazepam, there was a positive correlation between the performance on some tasks and the serum levels.

Andrewes et al. (1986) compared new referrals with epilepsy, well controlled on single drug therapy, with either phenytoin or carbamazepine and an untreated control group with respect to their performance on a number of cognitive tasks. These patients, who had well-controlled seizures, were tested at variable intervals after starting their medications, and they noticed significant differences between the groups in favour of carbamazepine. With the exception of a tracking task, patients on phenytoin performed consistently less well, these differences between phenytoin and carbamazepine being similar to those reported above.

Mattson et al. (1985) recently reported on a multicentre double-blind trial comparing the efficacy and toxicity of four anticonvulsant drugs all prescribed in monotherapy. These were carbmazepine, phenobarbitone, phenytoin and primidone, patients being newly assigned for treatment. Carbamazepine not only proved to be significantly better with regards to the total control of partial seizures when compared to phenobarbitone or primidone, but when the results of patients' testing on a cognitive battery were analysed, testing being carried out at one- three- and six-monthly intervals after initiation of treatment, carbamazepine was reported to have the least effect on a number of tasks including finger tapping, colour naming, a peg board test, a digit symbol substitution test, and discriminative reaction time. Phenytoin and phenobarbitone provided the worst scores, and correlations between deterioration and serum levels were noted (Smith et al., 1985; Chapter 6).

These data from several different centres, evaluating both volunteers and patients, suggest there are differences in the behavioural toxicity profile of the anticonvulsant drugs with regards to their impact on cognitive function. In all of the studies carbamazepine comes out as the drug with the least impact, while phenytoin, and where studied clonazepam, appear to have maximal effect. Although further information is required on other compounds, in particular phenobarbitone and ethosuximide, these data have important implications when considering choice of therapy for patients with seizure disorders.

Polytherapy

Although individual drugs may thus have a different impact with regards to cognitive function, polytherapy itself may be an important variable. Shorvon and Reynolds (1979) reduced polytherapy to monotherapy in 29 of 40 chronic epileptic patients, and reported an improvement in their mental state, commenting in particular on alertness, concentration, drive, mood and sociability. Withdrawal of phenobarbitone and phenytoin appears to be of most importance.

In institutionalized handicapped patients, the Milano Collaborative Group (1977) and Fischbacher (1982) have also reported beneficial effects on psychomotor performance by reducing medication in patients on polytherapy.

At the National Hospitals, changes in performance on a psychological test battery in patients on polytherapy have been examined in three groups whose anticonvulsant drugs have been altered in various ways. In the first group, 20 patients underwent reduction of polytherapy, their anticonvulsant drug prescriptions being approximately halved. In a second group, patients underwent reduction of medication but in addition were prescribed carbamazepine as a substitute for one or all of their treatments. Half of this group achieved carbamazepine monotherapy. The third group consisted of ten patients who did not have any anticonvulsant changes made and acted as a control group. Patients were seen on three occasions at three-monthly intervals, and following the first test session the medication changes were made. Psychological testing was carried out as noted above. The overall findings of these studies (Thompson and Trimble, 1982a) were that both groups undergoing treatment changes showed improvement in performance which were not seen in the patients on stable therapy. For the first group, improvements were most marked on measures of concentration and motor speed, and least marked on tests of memory. These benefits were generally not seen to be significant until the third treatment session, namely six months after the drug changes. Patients changing to carbamazepine either alone or in combination with some existing medication displayed even more widespread improvements on the test battery, with significant improvements of memory function. Further, changes in test performance were generally apparent at three months following the drug sessions and were maintained through to the six-month session.

In a more recent investigation, an attempt to replicate these findings in children has been carried out (Cull and Trimble, 1988; Chapter 8). In essence, although the results were less clearcut than the adult study, and a number of methodological reasons may explain this, these data also indicate that lowering the anticonvulsant prescription load of children improves cognitive performance, while increasing it has a deleterious effect on learning abilities. These data on both children and adults, using automated techniques to assess cognitive function, and following patients over a series of months, confirms clinical impressions and anecdotal reports that reduction of anticonvulsant drugs in patients with polytherapy is followed by beneficial cognitive effects.

BEHAVIOUR CHANGES

In contrast to cognitive function, which is measured using psychological tests, behaviour changes are usually assessed by giving patients rating scales which have previously been validated and standardized. As with the cognitive studies, in which a different profile of the drugs with regards to their detrimental and beneficial effects can be discerned, so it is with the behavioural effects. Thus, shortly following its introduction in the management of epilepsy, carbamazepine was reported to have psychotropic properties. Dalby (1975) reported that in 40 investigations on over 2000 patients a psychotropic effect with carbamazepine was seen in approximately 50%. Although he based his conclusions on largely uncontrolled reports and his own clinical experiences, more recently a number of controlled investigations in patients with epilepsy are available. Rajotte et al. (1967) noted a significant improvement in behaviour as measured on rating scales in a double-blind crossover trial in which carbamazepine was compared to phenytoin in chronic institutionalized epileptic patients. This occurred in spite of no changes of seizure frequency. Marjerrison et al. (1968), also using rating scales, compared carbamazepine to phenytoin and noted that patients were less retarded and less 'unhappy' on carbamazepine. Cereghino (1982) rated behaviour on a 53-item scale which was completed by ward attendants in patients who had their medication changed from regular prescriptions to carbamazepine, phenobarbitone or phenytoin. The behaviour of more patients deteriorated on phenytoin, and improvements were seen with both phenobarbitone and carbamazepine. Rodin et al. (1976) stabilized 40 patients on phenytoin and either primidone or carbamazepine. After a three-month period, those on carbamazepine were switched to primidone and vice versa. Using the Minnesota Multiphasic Personality Inventory, patients on primidone scored higher on the psychopathic deviant scale. Over time, clinically, patients became more depressed on the primidone and less so on carbamazepine. In a similarly designed study, Dodrill and Troupin (1977) compared carbamazepine to phenytoin over a four-month period using a double-blind crossover design, patients being randomly assigned. On the Minnesota Multiphasic Personality Inventory, every clinical scale favoured carbamazepine, statistically significant differences being noted for the F-scale which relates to feelings, attitudes and emotions.

With regards to the relationship of individual drugs to mood, it is interesting that there at least four studies in epileptic patients showing a significant negative relationship between serum levels of carbamazepine and scores on a mood or behaviour rating scale. Thus, Trimble and Corbett (1980), examining children on polytherapy, asked teachers and house parents to fill in the Rutter rating scales for the evaluation of behaviour. In this population, 42% were rated as having conduct disorders, the highest incidence of the latter was recorded in children on phenobarbitone, some 50% being affected. When only brighter children were examined (IQ >70), to minimize the influence of severe brain damage on the results, a significant negative correlation was noted between the behaviour deviancy score for conduct disorder and the serum levels of carbamazepine. This was in contrast to a positive correlation for phenobarbitone, the differences between phenobarbitone and carbamazepine being significant.

In adults, there are three studies showing a similar relationship. Robertson (Chapter 11) studied patients with depression and epilepsy who satisfied the Research Diagnostic Criteria for major depressive disorder. Patients who were taking phenobarbitone were more likely to record higher depression scores, and patients on carbamezepine rated themselves as less depressed, and had lower anxiety scores than those not receiving the drug. Significant negative correlations were found between trait anxiety scores and serum carbamazepine levels. Rodin and Schmaltz (1984) gave the Bear-Fedio inventory, a rating scale specifically designed for detection of behaviour disturbances in patients with epilepsy, to 148 patients and noted that carbamazepine serum levels were significantly inversely correlated with total score on the Bear-Fedio scale, and subscores for elation, philosophical interest, sense of destiny, altered sexuality and hypergraphia. Similar associated were not found for the other anticonvulsants. Finally, Andrewes et al. (1986) gave the Mood Adjective Check List to 42 patients, half of whom were started on monotherapy with phenytoin, the other half on monotherapy with carbamazepine. At follow-up they reported that the higher the serum level of carbamazepine, the lower the rating scale score was for anxiety, fatigue and depression.

These data are complemented by the results of a series of studies in which healthy volunteers were given anticonvulsant drugs over a two-week period in a double-blind crossover design briefly discussed above. In those studies, volunteers on phenytoin rated themselves as being more anxious, more tired and more depressed, significantly so for tiredness. On carbamazepine, changes in mood were minimal, but the direction of the changes suggested improvement.

Polytherapy

The anecdotal reports, e.g. those of Shorvon and Reynolds (1979), suggest that rationalization of polytherapy brings improvement of mood. In the investigations of Thompson and Trimble (1982a, b) two groups of patients had rationalization of their polytherapy carried out, in one carbamazepine being substituted for one or all of the drugs that the patients were receiving. A third group acted as a control group. Patients were given the Mood Adjective Check List, and the Middlesex Hospital Questionnaire, in order to assess changes of mood. Assessments were carried out at three months and six months following the change of medication. The control group showed no changes of mood, while the group who had their polytherapy rationalized showed significant improvements on rating scales of mood in particular for anxiety and depression. Following the carbamazepine substitution, patients rated themselves as less anxious and more lively during the follow-up period. With regards to depression, when patients were divided into those with high or low initial (prechange) depression scores, those with the higher scores showed significant improvements following the change to carbamazepine.

SUMMARY AND CONCLUSIONS

A summary of the data derived from investigations reported in this chapter are shown in Table 1. In brief, it has been possible to discern in the literature two aspects which have been investigated in relationship to behavioural toxicity profiles of anticonvulsants. The first relates to cognitive function, the ability of patients to carry out psychological tasks speedily and correctly, as opposed to behaviour, namely assessment of mood and personality. With regards to cognitive function, most studies contrast the more detrimental effects of phenytoin with the least detrimental effects of carbamazepine, drugs such as sodium valproate appearing to hold an intermediate position. Phenobarbitone and clonazepam are more likely to be associated with the phenytoin spectrum of activity, although further investigations of these drugs are warranted.

In contrast, with the behavioural studies, carbamazepine can be more effectively contrasted with phenobarbitone. Several studies, and many anecdotal reports, suggest that carbamazepine is psychotropic, while phenobarbitone may exacerbate or even precipitate affective disturbances in adults and conduct disturbances in children. The relationship to serum levels with regards to the behavioural profile of carbamazepine is striking. Even stronger evidence for the psychotropic effects of this drug emerges from the growing literature of its effective use in non-epileptic patients with bipolar affective disorder who receive carbamazepine, either acutely in the management of mania, or for the prophylaxis of manic depressive illness (Post, 1985). Although it is not suggested that all of the cognitive and behavioural problems that patients with epilepsy suffer from are related to anticonvulsant drugs, and a number of other variables are urgently in need of further investigation in their own right, it is suggested that these data have importance for the management of epilepsy, particularly when patients or their relatives complain of such problems.

Table 1. Summary of the effects of anticonvulsants on cognitive function and behaviour

	Behaviour	Cognitive function
Carbamazepine	Minimal	Minimal
Clonazepam	Impairs	Impairs
Ethosuximide	?	?
Phenobarbitone	Impairs	Minimal
Phenytoin	Minimal	Impairs
Sodium valproate	Minimal	?

ACKNOWLEDGEMENTS

The author wishes to acknowledge the generous financial support of the Thorn Epilepsy Research Fund, the Brain Research Trust, the Raymond Way Memorial Trust and the Clarkson Trust in relationship to investigations carried out at the Institute of Neurology quoted in this chapter.

REFERENCES

ANDREWES, D.G., BULLEN, J.G., TOMLINSON, L., ELWES, R.D.C. and REYNOLDS, E.H. (1986) A comparative study of the cognitive effects of phenytoin and carbamazepine in new referrals with epilepsy. *Epilepsia*, **27**, 128–134.

CEREGHINO, J.J. (1982) Carbamazepine. In WOODBURY, D.M., PENRY, J.K. and PIPPENGER, C.E. (eds) *Antiepileptic Drugs*. New York, Raven Press, pp. 507–519.

CULL, C.A. and TRIMBLE, M.R. (1985) Anticonvulsant benzodiazepines and performance. International Congress and Symposium Series of the Royal Society of Medicine No.74, pp. 121–128.

CULL, C.A. and TRIMBLE, M.R. (1988) Changes in drug regime and cognitive function in children with epilepsy. In preparation.

DALBY, M.A. (1975) Behavioural effects of carbamazepine. In PENRY J.K. and DALY, D.D. (eds) *Advances in Neurology II*. New York, Raven Press, pp. 331–344.

DODRILL, C.B. and TROUPIN, A.S. (1977) Psychotropic effect of carbamazepine in epilepsy. A double-blind comparison with phenytoin. *Neurology*, **27**, 1023–1028.

FISCHBACHER, E. (1982) Effect of reduction of anticonvulsants on well being. *Br. Med. J*. 423–425.

MARJERRISON, G. et al. (1968) Carbamazepine: Behavioural, anticonvulsant and EEG effects in chronically hospitalised epileptics. *Dis. Nerv. Syst.*, **29**, 133–136.

MATTSON, R.H. et al. (1985) Comparison of carbamazepine, phenobarbital, phenytoin and primidone in partial and secondarily generalised tonic-clonic seizures. *New Eng. J. Med.*, **313**, 145–151.

Milano Collaborative Group of Studies on Epilepsy (1977) Long-term intensive monitoring in the difficult patient. In GARDNER-THORPE et al. (eds), *Antiepileptic Drug Monitoring*. Tunbridge Wells, Pitman, pp. 197–213.

POST, R.M., UHDE, T.W., JOFFE, R.T., ROY-BYRNE, P.P. and KELLHER, C. (1985) Anti-convulsant drugs in psychiatric illness. In TRIMBLE, M.R. (ed) *The psychopharmacology of Epilepsy*. Chichester, John Wiley & Sons, pp. 141–171.

RAJOTTE, P. et al. (1967) Propiétés antiépileptiques et psychotropes de la carbamazepine. *Union Medicale, Canada*, **96**, 1200–1206.

RODIN, E.A. et al. (1976) A comparison of the effectiveness of primidone versus carbamazepine in epileptic outpatients. *J.Nerv.Ment.Dis.*, **163**, 41–46.

RODIN, E.A. and SCHMALTZ, S. (1984) The Bear–Fedio personality inventory and temporal lobe epilepsy. *Neurology*, **34**, 591–596.

SHORVON, S. and REYNOLDS, E.H. (1979) Reduction in polypharmacy for epilepsy. *Br.Med.J.*, **2**, 1023–1025.

SMITH, D.B., CRAFT, R.B., VA Cooperative Study Group (1985) Differential neurotoxicity of four major anticonvulsants. *Ann.Neurol.*, **18**, 119.

THOMPSON, P.J. and TRIMBLE, M.R. (1981) Clobazam and cognitive functions. Royal Society of Medicine International Congress and Symposium Series. London, Academic Press, pp. 33–38.

THOMPSON, P.J. and TRIMBLE, M.R. (1982a) Anticonvulsant drugs and cognitive functions. *Epilepsia*, **33**, 531–534.

THOMPSON, P.J. and TRIMBLE, M.R. (1982b) Comparative effects of anticonvulsant drugs on cognitive functioning. *Br. J. Clin. Pract*, **18** (suppl), 154–156.

THOMPSON, P.J. and TRIMBLE, M.R. (1983) Anticonvulsant serum levels; relationship to impairments of cognitive functioning. *J. Neurol Neurosurg. Psychiat.*, **46**, 227–233.

THOMPSON, R.J., HUPPERT, F.A. and TRIMBLE, M.R. (1981) Phenytoin and cognitive functions: effects on normal volunteers and implications for epilepsy. *Br.J.Clin. Psychol.*, **20**, 155–162.

TRIMBLE, M.R. (1985) Psychiatric and psychological aspects of epilepsy. In PORTER, R.J. and MORSELLI, P.L. (eds) *The Epilepsies*. London, Butterworths, pp. 322–355.

TRIMBLE, M.R. and CORBETT, J.A. (1980) Behavioural and cognitive disturbances in epileptic children. *Irish Medical J.*, **73**, (suppl), 21–28.

TRIMBLE, M.R. and REYNOLDS, E.H. (1976) Anticonvulsant drugs and mental symptoms. A review. *Psychol. Med.*, **6**, 169–178.

11

Epilepsy and mood

MARY M. ROBERTSON
The Middlesex Hospital, London

Cassius: But soft, I pray you. What, did Caesar swoon?
Casca: He fell down in the market-place, and foamed at the mouth and was
speechless.
Brutus: 'Tis very like. He hath the falling sickness . . .
Casca: I know not what you mean by that, but I am sure
Caesar fell down . . .
Marry, before he fell down, when he perceived the common herd was glad
he refused the crown, he plucked me ope his doublet, and offered then to
cut his throat.

Julius Caesar, I, ii, William Shakespeare

INTRODUCTION

It seems there is no doubt that Julius Caesar suffered from epilepsy; moreover,
it may be argued that while in a peri-ictal state, just prior to the seizure
described, his mood was dysphoric, even amounting to a peri-ictal depressive
episode, in that he requested that he might die, by having his throat cut.
Disorders of mood are commonly associated with epilepsy. This chapter will
consider, in the main, depression, but will also touch on anxiety, mania and
elation.

Depression has been associated with epilepsy since some of the earliest
medical recordings. Thus, Hippocrates thought epilepsy and melancholia were
closely related when he commented 'melancholics ordinarily become epileptics
and epileptics melancholics: of these two states what determines the preference
is the direction the malady takes: if it bears upon the body, epilepsy; if upon the
intelligence, melancholy' (Lewis, 1934). Many others in the early literature
also noted a link between depression and epilepsy (Griesinger, 1857; White,
1900; Barham, 1907; Baugh, 1908; Jones, 1912). In keeping with one of the

classifications of psychiatric disorders in association with epilepsy, the relationship may be defined as peri-ictal (directly related to the ictus) or interictal (in which the psychiatric concomitants are chronic and not directly related to the ictal electrical disturbances).

PERI-ICTAL DEPRESSION

There are not many documentations of this particular condition, but nevertheless lowered mood around the ictus has been recognized for some time by physicians (Reynolds, 1861; Mulder and Daly, 1952; Weil, 1955, 1959; Williams, 1956). Characteristically, the alteration of mood lasts longer than an aura or postictal automatism, and it can have dangerous consequences, as evidenced by Betts (1982) who reported a patient who cut his throat during an ictal depressive state. Julius Caesar, as we have seen, requested in a pre-ictal state that his throat be cut: this was not done, but Caesar, not listening to the prophetical warnings of the soothsayer surrounding the Ides of March, entered the marketplace and was consequently murdered by his senators. Prolonged depressive mood swings have been recorded during status epilepticus (Wells, 1975; Lim et al., 1986), petit mal status (Tucker and Forster, 1950; Jaffe, 1963) and partial seizure status (Henriksen, 1973). Two patients who presented with depression, and who were investigated, were shown to be in temporal lobe status (Robertson, 1986): both had previous depressive episodes requiring treatment. Others (Gupta et al., 1983) have described affective symptomatology as the most common aura in patients attending neurology clinics, while Greenberg et al. (1984) described four patients with complex partial seizures who became preoccupied with death during their seizures, which were accompanied by periods of anxiety, terror, fear, agitation and depression. Several others have noted ictal fear (Hermann and Chabria, 1980; Ficol et al., 1984) and other dysphoric episodes shown subsequently to be ictally related (Graham and Freeman, 1982; Blanchet and Frommer, 1986).

INTERICTAL DEPRESSION

Although many refer to 'depression' in association with epilepsy, few studies have defined the word precisely, some clearly referring to depressive symptomatology, while others would probably be implying depressive illness. Bearing in mind the controversy surrounding the classification of depression (Kendell, 1976), an attempt will be made to examine interictal depressed moods.

No studies have directly addressed the question as to whether depression occurs more frequently in people with epilepsy compared to other conditions, but conclusions may be drawn indirectly from the results of investigations using standardized rating scales. Thus, many studies employing the Minnesota

Multiphasic Personality Inventory (MMPI) have indicated that depression scores are raised in people with epilepsy (Modlin, 1960; Guerrant et al., 1962; Klove and Doehring, 1962; Meier and French, 1965; Matthews and Kløve, 1968; Mignone et al., 1970; Glass and Mattson, 1973), with special reference to those with psychomotor/temporal lobe epilepsy (Stevens, 1975; Rodin et al., 1976; Hermann et al., 1982; Dikmen et al., 1983). Other investigators, employing the Present State Examination (Standage and Fenton, 1975), the Bear–Fedio Personal Inventory (Bear and Fedio, 1977), the Crown Crisp Experiential Index (Trimble and Perez, 1982a, b; Kogeorgos et al., 1982; Fenton, 1986), the Clinical Interview Schedule (Edeh and Toone, 1985) and the Standard Psychiatric Interview (Brown et al., 1986) have all found that patients with epilepsy have had higher depression scores than controls. Some have noted that the scores obtained are similar to those found in psychiatric outpatients (Trimble and Perez, 1982a, b) but may not be particularly high for a general hospital outpatient population (Brown et al., 1986). This is in contrast to the findings of Angelis and Vizioli (1983) who found that patients with epilepsy scored no higher than patients with syncopal attacks and chronic non-neurological diseases on two depression rating scales.

The question as to whether those patients with temporal lobe epilepsy/complex partial seizures are more prone to depression is largely unanswered. Brown et al. (1986) found that those with temporal lobe epilepsy complained of more irritability and impaired concentration and were rated as more depressed and 'slowed up', disagreeing with Trimble and Perez (1982a, b) who found no relationship between type of epilepsy and depression.

Whitman et al. (1984) analysed MMPI data on ten studies of patients with epilepsy embracing 809 subjects, 22 studies of patients with neurological disorders totalling 870 people, and 15 studies of groups of patients with non-neurological disorders consisting of 1107 subjects with problems as diverse as cardiac disease, asthma, renal disease, burns and arthritis. They used a recognized MMPI sequential diagnostic system to analyse the profiles of the patients and results showed that those with epilepsy ran a higher risk for psychopathology than members of the general population. However, no increase of psychopathology was found in patients with epilepsy compared to those with other chronic disorders, and no difference was found between patients with temporal lobe and generalized epilepsy. In fact, patients with neurological illness were found to be at significantly greater risk compared to people with epilepsy and other chronic illnesses, although it was agreed that the neurological group was heterogeneous. Dodrill and Batzel (1986) performed a similar type of investigation on 17 studies evaluating interictal behaviour using standardized objective measures including the MMPI. However, there was only partial agreement with Whitman et al. (1984); they concluded that persons with epilepsy exhibited more emotional and psychiatric problems than normal controls, but to a similar degree as patients with other neurological disorders.

They also suggested that increased emotional and psychiatric problems were not found in people with temporal lobe epilepsy compared to other types of epilepsy but that there was a subgroup of patients who did demonstrate behavioural traits, supposedly characteristic. Dodrill and Batzel (1986), however, suggested that the number of seizure types was far more relevant to psychopathology than was the particular seizure type.

Several clinical investigations (Dominian et al., 1963; Currie et al., 1971; Taylor, 1972; Betts, 1974; Serafetinides, 1975; Gunn, 1977; Toone and Driver, 1980; Mellor et al., 1974; Pazzangia and Frank Pazzangia, 1976) have reported depression to be common in both adult and child patients with epilepsy.

Schofield and Duane (1986) investigated psychopathology amongst referrals to a neurological liaison service and reported that the most common conditions were epilepsy, Parkinsonism and cervical spondylosis. Of the 30 patients with epilepsy, 43% of those who qualified for a diagnosis had a depressive illness. Thus, so far it can be seen that, regardless of the source of referral, namely psychiatric, neurological or general practice, most investigations are fairly consistent in demonstrating that depressive symptomatology and possibly depressive illness is common in patients with epilepsy.

Several studies have explored specific aspects of the depression seen in people with epilepsy. Several authors have noted a decrease in fit frequency prior to the onset of the depressive illness (Dongier, 1959–60; Flor-Henry, 1969; Betts, 1974; Standage and Fenton, 1975). Flor-Henry (1969) suggested that when a patient had a combination of temporal lobe epilepsy and affective psychosis, a non-dominant abnormality was likely to be found, but this association has only been reaffirmed by a few subsequent authors (for review, see Trimble and Robertson, 1987). Other studies have thus specifically investigated the laterality hypothesis. Nielsen and Kristensen (1981) evaluated 42 patients with temporal lobe epilepsy (L=23, R=19) using the Bear–Fedio Personality Inventory, and left-sided foci patients scored significantly higher than right-sided subjects on the traits depression and emotionality combined. Perini and Mendius (1983; 1984) evaluated 41 patients with complex partial seizures (20 with left and 21 with right temporal lobe foci) and 38 matched control subjects using standardized rating scales, and left-sided patients scored higher than both right-sided patients and controls on measures of depression. Camfield et al. (1984) assessed 27 children with lateralized temporal lobe epilepsy (14=right, 13=left), with parents completing a personality inventory for children: no right–left differences were found on depression or anxiety scores. Brandt et al. (1985) tested the laterality hypothesis, and failed to support the notion that sadness/mood were associated with right temporal lobe disturbance.

Roy (1979) evaluated 42 patients admitted to hospital for investigation and treatment of their epilepsy using the Hamilton Depression Rating Scale (HDRS). He divided them into two groups: 23 with depressive symptoms

(HDRS score 9 or above) and 19 with an HDRS score below 9. Results showed no differences in mean ages of the groups or the age of onset or duration of epilepsy, while no difference was reported between affective symptoms and type of epilepsy. Significantly more in the groups with depressive symptoms had a past history of neurotic disorder than those without. In a survey of psychiatric day and inpatients with epilepsy, Palia and Harper (1986) judged 17 as clinically depressed, with a mean HDRS score of 21 and a mean Beck Depression Inventory (BDI) score of 32. Twelve were classified as non-endogenous on the Newcastle Scale. Eighty-eight per cent of the group were female and the depressed patients had experienced significantly more life events during the three months prior to the assessment. The depressed group also had a significantly greater past history of depression, deliberate drug overdose and self-harm. Electroencephalographic studies were used to test the laterality hypothesis, failing to support it.

Two investigations have examined the phenomenology of depressive illness in people with epilepsy, using entry diagnostic criteria and standardized rating scales, in addition to exploring possible relationships between the two conditions. Mendez et al. (1986) compared 20 depressed epileptics with 20 depressed individuals without epilepsy, all of whom satisfied DSM III criteria for major depression and had similar mean scores on the HDRS (21.7%; 24.7%, respectively). Results of analysis of data showed that male patients predominated in both groups, and equal numbers of patients in each group had made previous suicidal attempts. More control than index patients had a family history of depression, while more index patients had psychotic features. No associations were reported between depression and seizure frequency or the duration of the depression and serum anticonvulsant dosages or levels. Focal changes on the electroencephalogram were evident in 15 patients, of which ten were on the left, nine being in the temporal area.

Robertson et al. (1987) assessed 66 patients who fulfilled epilepsy criteria, the Research Diagnostic Criteria for major depressive disorder and who scored over 12 on the HDRS. Sixteen patients had a family history of psychopathology, with depression being the most common diagnosis. Forty-three patients had a past history of depression, while 13 were psychotic as defined by mood congruent hallucinations or delusions. Only two patients had a history of bipolar disorder. Half the patients were receiving two anticonvulsants agents, 27 being on monotherapy with carbamazepine and phenytoin being the most prescribed drugs. Forty-five patients had complex partial seizures (25 secondarily generalized), nine had secondarily generalized seizures, eight had primary generalized seizures and one was unclassified due to insufficient information. Electroencephalographic examinations were performed on the patients and matched controls, and the majority showed temporal lobe abnormalities. Statistical analysis showed no significant differences between patient and control groups: among those with temporal lobe abnormalities there was a bias to the left, which was most marked in the patient group. The severity of the depression was moderate on the HDRS, BDI and Levine-Pilowsky Questionnaire (LPD), while 28 (42.4%) were rated as endogenous on the Newcastle Scale and 25 (37.9%) on the LPD. Attendant features of the depression were high state anxiety, high neuroticism and high hostility, especially the intropunitive scores of self-criticism and guilt. The duration of epilepsy correlated significantly with the severity of the depression and an association was found between complex partial seizures and a past history of depression. No other significant relationships were found between depression and epilepsy variables. Thus, the type, severity and features of depression were not influenced by the age of onset of epilepsy, the type of epilepsy, the site of a focal lesion or seizure frequency. An exception was the effect of anticonvulsants on mood, in that patients receiving phenobarbitone were more depressed than those not receiving the drug, while patients on carbamazepine were less depressed and had lower trait anxiety. There were, moreover, significant negative correlations between trait anxiety scores and both carbamazepine dose and level.

SUICIDE AND PARASUICIDE

Germane to any discussion about depression is the problem of suicide. Patients with affective disorder are particularly at risk, with patients treated for manic-depressive psychosis and depressive illness having approximately 30 times the risk of death by suicide compared to the general population. In people with epilepsy, suicide and attempted suicide are also common, in that the risk for suicide is four to five times greater than that of the general population (Barraclough, 1981; Matthews and Barabas, 1981; Wannamaker, 1983), while those with temporal lobe epilepsy have an increased risk of 25 times the expected (Barraclough, 1981). Two studies have documented a 5–7 per cent increase in self-poisoning in people with epilepsy (Mackay, 1979; Hawton, 1980).

TREATMENT

Psychotherapy is important in people with depression, especially if they have epilepsy as well, and may take the form of supportive therapy or a combination of formal therapy (such as cognitive or behavioural approaches) and antidepressants which is shown to be highly effective (Weissman, 1981).

Assessment and rationalization of the patient's anticonvulsant regimen is also important. An improvement in mental state has been found with reduction of polypharmacy (Thompson and Trimble, 1982; Giordani et al., 1983; Albright and Bruni, 1985). If monotherapy is appropriate, carbamazepine would be the drug of choice as it has been shown to be antidepressant in depressed people without epilepsy (Folks et al., 1982), as having a prophylactic effect in manic depressive illness (Ballenger and Post, 1980; Okuma et al., 1981) and having a psychotropic effect in people with epilepsy (Dalby, 1971; Dodrill and Troupin, 1977; Rodin and Schmaltz, 1984; Robertson et al., 1987).

The role of antidepressants in people with epilepsy has to be addressed with several issues in mind; namely the effects of antidepressants on the seizure threshold, antidepressant–anticonvulsant interactions and the efficacy of the antidepressant in the particular setting. It is well known that virtually all non-monoamine oxidase inhibitor antidepressants lower the seizure threshold (Trimble, 1978), but to varying degrees. Taking data from several sources such as the Committee on the Safety of Medicines (CSM), (Edwards, 1985), experimental studies (Trimble et al., 1977; Jobe et al., 1984; Luchins et al., 1984), studies on patient populations (Crome and Newman, 1977; Bowdan, 1983; Lefkowitz et al., 1985; Hohly and Martin, 1986) and recently acquired information (Edwards and Glen-Bott, 1984; Krijzer et al., 1984; Cilasun et al., 1986), and treatment reports (Ojemann et al., 1983; Robertson and Trimble, 1985) into account, it would seem that the antidepressants most likely to be implicated with seizures are maprotiline, minaserin, trazodone and clomipramine, while drugs which are less likely to be associated are doxepin, fluvoxamine, viloxazine, protriptyline, butriptyline and the MAOIs: viloxazine should probably be avoided, however, because of its potential to cause anticonvulsant toxicity.

MANIA AND ELATION

Manic psychoses in the context of epilepsy are, in contrast, rarely reported. Wolf (1982) reviewed the literature and found only nine case-studies of mania in people with epilepsy. He reported an additional six patients with manic syndromes: of these one patient had generalized epilepsy, while five had temporal lobe epilepsy. In three of the patients the manic states were part of the epileptic process, as they were closely related in time to the seizures. Of these, one had a postictal psychosis, while two were associated with decreased seizure frequency, one showing 'forced normalization'. Toone et al. (1982) conducted a retrospective investigation on 69 patients with a combined diagnosis of epilepsy and psychosis and, of these, only three showed evidence of bipolarity. Robertson et al. (1987) took past psychiatric histories on 66 depressed epileptic patients and only two had bipolar illness. Roberts et al. (1982) describe a further patient with epilepsy and a manic-depressive presentation. Recently Barczak et al. (1988) reported three cases of short-lived hypomania following complex partial seizures. All these fulfilled DSM III criteria for hypomania, and were all similar in that they were middle-aged men with right-sided (non-dominant) temporal lobe epilepsy who became hypomanic following an increase in their seizures and who exhibited affect-laden hallucinations and delusions with a religious theme. The patients' mental state was further characterized by clear consciousness and returned to normal with adequate seizure control. One possible reason for the protection of epileptic patients from manic swings is that most will be on anticonvulsant medication including phenobarbitone, sodium valproate and carbamazepine, all of which have been shown to affect mood (Robertson et al., 1987; Post et al., 1985; Emrich et al., 1984), albeit in different ways. Elation, too, has been described in people with epilepsy, but only in the context of patients with hypergraphia, hyper-religiosity and déjà vu experiences (Roberts et al., 1982) and is not frequently encountered.

DISCUSSION AND CONCLUSIONS

From the review it is concluded that mood disorders occur frequently in people with epilepsy, but that this applies predominantly to anxiety, depressive symptomatology and depressive illness; mania and elation appear to occur rarely, although the apparent infrequency may, in part, be due to lack of documentation of cases. With regards to depressive symptoms, several studies using standardized rating scales have found the depression scores to range from moderate to severe and to compare favourably to studies on depressed patients without epilepsy. Although only two investigations specifically addressed depressive illness in the context of epilepsy, employing currently accepted diagnostic criteria, many of the patients included in the studies would probably qualify for a depressive illness. There seems to be agreement on several issues. A number of variables have been suggested with regard to the pathogenesis of the depression, and several predisposing or provoking factors include genetic endowment, patients' fears, social stigmatization, adverse life events and a past history of depressive illness. Moreover, the phenomenology of the depression does not, on the whole, seem linked with epilepsy variables. Anticonvulsants can however affect the mental state, and the longer the duration of epilepsy the more severe the depression. The majority of studies implicated the left hemisphere, with hints that temporal lobe/complex partial seizure patients are more vulnerable.

REFERENCES

ALBRIGHT, P. and BRUNI, J. (1985) Reduction of polypharmacy in epileptic patients. *Arch. Neurol.*, **42**, 797–799.

ANGELIS, G. DE and VIZIOLI, R. (1983) Epilepsy and depression. In *Advances in Epileptology XIVth Epilepsy International Symposium*, pp. 203–206 (eds M. PARSONAGE, R.H.E. GRANT, A. CRAIG and A.A.J. WARD), Raven Press, New York.

BALLENGER, J.C. and POST, R.M. (1980) Carbamazepine (Tegretol) in manic-depressive illness: a new treatment. *Am. J. Psych.*, **137**, 782–790.

BARCZAK, P., EDMUNDS, E. and BETTS, T. (1988) Hypomania following complex partial seizures. *Br. J. Psych.*, **152**, 137–139.

BARHAM, G.R. (1907) Notes on the management and treatment of the epileptic insane, with special reference to the NaCl-free (or hypo-chlorisation) diet. *J. Ment. Sci.*, **53**, 361–367.

BARRACLOUGH, B. (1981) Suicide and epilepsy. In *Epilepsy and Psychiatry*, pp. 72–76 (eds E.H. REYNOLDS and M.R. TRIMBLE). Churchill-Livingstone, Edinburgh.

BAUGH, L.D.H. (1908) Observations on insane epileptics treated under hospital principles. *J. Ment. Sci.*, **54**, 518–528.

BEAR, D.M. and FEDIO, P. (1977) Quantitative analysis of interictal behavior in temporal lobe epilepsy. *Arch. Neurol.*, **34**, 454–467.

BETTS, T.A. (1974) A follow-up study of a cohort of patients with epilepsy admitted to psychiatric care in an English city. In *Proceedings of the Hans Berger Centenary Symposium*, pp. 326–338 (eds P. HARRIS and C. MAWDSLEY). Churchill Livingstone, Edinburgh.

BETTS, T.A. (1982) Psychiatry and epilepsy: part one. In *A Textbook of Epilepsy*, 2nd edition pp. 227–270 (eds J. LAIDLAW and A. RICHENS). Churchill-Livingstone, Edinburgh.

BLANCHET, P. and FROMMER, G.P. (1986) Mood change preceding epileptic seizures. *J. Nerv. Ment. Dis.*, **174**, 471–476.

BOWDAN, N.D. (1983) Seizure possibly caused by trazodone HCL. *Am. J. Psych.* **140**, 642.

BRANDT, J., SEIDMAN, L.J. and KOHL, D. (1985) Personality characteristics of epileptic patients: a controlled study of generalised and temporal lobe cases. *J. Clin. Exper. Neuropsychology*, **7**, 25–38.

BROWN, S.W., MCGOWAN, M.E.L. and REYNOLDS, E.H. (1986) The influence of seizure type and medication on psychiatric symptoms in epileptic patients. *Br. J. Psych.*, **148**, 300–304.

CAMFIELD, P.R., GATES, R., RONEN, G., CAMFIELD, C., FERGUSON, A. and MAC-DONALD, G.W. (1984) Comparison of cognitive ability, personality profile and school success in epileptic children with pure right versus left temporal lobe EEG foci. *Ann. Neurol.*, **15**, 122–126.

CILASUN, J., EDWARDS, J.G. and SEDGWICK, E.M. (1986) Electroencephalographic changes during treatment with clovoxamine fumarate. *Neuropharmacology*, **25**, 665–667.

CROME, P. and NEWMAN, B. (1977) Poisoning with maprotiline and mianserin. *Brit. Med. J.*, **ii**, 260.

CURRIE, S., HEATHFILED, K.W.G., HENSON, R.A. and SCOTT, D.F. (1971) Clinical course and prognosis of temporal lobe epilepsy: a survey of 666 patients. *Brain*, **94**, 173–190.

DALBY, M.A. (1971) Antiepileptic and psychotropic effect of carbamazepine (Tegretol) in the treatment of psychomotor epilepsy. *Epilepsia*, **12**, 325–333.

DIKMEN, S., HERMANN, B.P., WILENSKY, A.J. and RAINWATER, G. (1983) Validity of the Minnesota Multiphasic Personality Inventory (MMPI) to psychopathology in patients with epilepsy. *J. Nerv. Ment. Dis.*, **171**, 114–122.

DODRILL, C.B. and BATZEL, L.W. (1986) Interictal behavioral features of patients with epilepsy. *Epilepsia*, **27** (Suppl 2), S64–S76.

DODRILL, C.B. and TROUPIN, A.S. (1977) Psychotropic effects of carbamazepine in epilepsy: a double-blind comparison with phenytoin. *Neurology*, **27**, 1023–1028.

DOMINIAN, J., SERAFETINIDES, E.A. and DEWHURST, M. (1963) A follow-up study of late onset epilepsy: II: psychiatric and social findings. *Brit. Med. J.*, **1**, 431–435.

DONGIER, S. (1959/1960) Statistical study of clinical and electroencephalographic manifestations of 536 psychotic episodes occurring in 516 epileptics between clinical seizures. *Epilepsia*, **1**, 117–142.

EDEH, J. and TOONE, B.K. (1985) Antiepileptic therapy, folate deficiency and psychiatric morbidity: a general practice survey, *Epilepsia*, **26**, 434–440.

EDWARDS, J.G. (1985) Antidepressants and seizures: epidemiological and clinical aspects. In *The Psychopharmacology of Epilepsy*, pp. 119–139 (ed. M.R. TRIMBLE), John Wiley & Sons, Chichester, 119–139.

EDWARDS, J.G. and GLEN-BOTT, M. (1984) Does viloxazine have epileptic properties? *J. Neurol. Neurosurg. Psychiatry*, **47**, 960–964.

EMRICH, H.M., DOSE, N., VON ZERSSEN, D. (1984) Action of sodium valproate and of oxcarbazepine in patients with affective disorders. In *Anticonvulsants in Affective Disorders*, pp. 45–55 (eds H.M. EMRICH, T. OKUMA and A.A. MULLER), Excerpta Medica, Amsterdam.

FENTON, G.W. (1986) Minor psychiatric morbidity in people with epilepsy: evidence for a gender difference. Presented at the Annual Meeting of the Royal College of Psychiatrists, 8–10th July, 1986, Southampton, United Kingdom.

FICOL, M., RAMANI, V. and HERRON, C. (1984) Episodic fear in epilepsy. *Epilepsia*, **25**, 669–670.

FLOR-HENRY, P. (1969) Psychosis and temporal lobe epilepsy: a controlled investigation. *Epilepsia*, **10**, 363–395.

FOLKS, D.G., KING, L.D., DOWDY, S.B., PETRIE, W.N., JACK, R.A., KOOMEN, J.C., SWENSON, B.R. and EDWARDS, P. (1982) Carbamazepine treatment of selected affectively disordered inpatients. *Am. J. Psych.*, **139**, 115–117.

GIORDANI, B., SACKELLARES, J.C., MILLER, S., BERENT, S., SUTULA, T., SEIDENBERG, M., BOLL, T.J., O'LEARY, D. and DREIFUSS, F.E. (1983) Improvement in neuropsychological performance in patients with refractory seizures after intensive diagnostic and therapeutic intervention. *Neurology*, **33**, 489–493.

GLASS, D.H. and MATTSON, R.H. (1973) Psychopathology and emotional precipitation of seizures in temporal lobe and nontemporal lobe epileptics. Proceedings of the 81st Annual Convention of the Americal Psychological Association, **8**, 425–426.

GRAHAM, B. and FREEMAN, F.R. (1982) Continuous psychomotor seizures presenting as longstanding mental illness. *Southern Medical Journal*, **75**, 505–506.

GREENBERG, D.B., HOCHBERG, F.H. and MURRAY, G.B. (1984) The theme of death in complex partial seizures. *Am. J. Psych.*, **141**, 1587–1589.

GRIESINGER, W. (1857) *Mental Pathology and Therapeutics*. Translated by Lockhart, Robertson and Rutherford J. New Sydenham Society, London.

GUERRANT, J., ANDERSON, W.W., FISCHER, A., WEINSTEIN, M.R., JAROS, R.M. and DESKINS, A. (1962) *Personality in Epilepsy*. Charles C. Thomas: Springfield, Ill.

GUNN, J. (1977) *Epileptics in Prison*. Academic Press, London.

GUPTA, A.K., JEAVONS, P.M., HUGHES, R.C. and COVANIS, A. (1983) Aura in temporal lobe epilepsy and electroencephalographic correlation. *J. Neurol. Neurosurg. Psychiatry*, **46**, 1079–1083.

HAWTON, K., FAGG, J. and MARSACK, P. (1980) Association between epilepsy and attempted suicide. *J. Neurol. Neurosurg. Psychiatry*, **43**, 168–170.

HENRIKSEN, G.F. (1973) Status epilepticus partialis with fear as clinical expression: report of a case and ictal EEG findings. *Epilepsia*, **14**, 39–46.

HERMANN, B.P. and CHABRIA, S. (1980) Interictal psychopathology in patients with ictal fear: examples of sensory-limbic hyperconnection? *Arch. Neurol.*, **37**, 667–668.

HERMANN, B.P., DIKMEN, S., SCHWARTZ, M.S. and KARNES, W.E. (1982) Interictal psychopathology in patients with ictal fear: a quantitative investigation. *Neurology*, **32**, 7–11.

HOHLY, E.K. and MARTIN, R.L. (1986) Increased seizure duration during ECT with Trazodone administration. *Am. J. Psychiat.*, **143**, 1326.

JAFFE, R. (1963) Ictal behaviour disturbance as the only manifestation of seizure disorder. *J. Nerv. Ment. Dis.*, **134**, 470–476.

JOBE, P.C., WOODS, T.W. and DAILEY, J.W. (1984) Pro-convulsant and anticonvulsant affects of tricyclic antidepressants in genetically epilepsy-prone rats. In *Advances in Epileptology*: 15th Epilepsy International Symposium, pp. 187–191 (eds. R.J. PORTER, R.J. MATTSON, A.A. WARD and M. DAM), Raven Press, New York.

JONES, R. (1912) The relation of epilepsy to insanity and its treatment. *Practitioner*, 89, 772–792.

KENDELL, R.E. (1976) The classification of depressions: a review of contemporary confusion., *Br. J. Psych.*, 129, 15–28.

KLØVE, H. and DOEHRING, D.G. (1962) MMPI in epileptic groups with differential etiology. *J. Clin. Psychol.*, 18, 149–153.

KOGEORGOS, J., FONAGY, P. and SCOTT, D.F. (1982) Psychiatric symptom patterns of chronic epileptics attending a neurological clinic: a controlled investigation, *Br. J. Psych.*, 140, 236–243.

KRIJZER, F., SNELDER, N. and BRADFORD, D. (1984) Comparison of the (pro) convulsive properties of fluvoxamine and clovoxamine with eight other antidepressants in the animal model. *Neuropsychobiology*, 12, 249–254.

LEFKOWITZ, D., KILGO, G. and LEE, S. (1985) Seizures and Trazodone therapy. *Arch. Gen. Psych.*, 42, 523.

LEWIS, A.J. (1934) Melancholia: a historical review. *J. Ment. Sci.*, 80, 1–42.

LIM, J., YAGNIK, P., SCHRAEDER, P. and WHEELER, S. (1986) Ictal catatonia as a manifestation of nonconvulsive status epilepticus, *J. Neurol. Neurosurg. Psychiatry*, 49, 833–836.

LUCHINS, D.J., OLIVER, A.P. and WYATT, R.J. (1984) Seizures with antidepressants: an in vitro technique to assess relative risk. *Epilepsia*, 25, 25–32.

MACKAY, A. (1979) Self-poisoning – a complication of epilepsy, *Br. J. Psychiat.*, 134, 277–282.

MATTHEWS, C.H.G. and KLØVE, H. (1968) MMPI performances in major motor, psychomotor and mixed seizure classifications of known and unknown etiology. *Epilepsia*, 9, 43–53.

MATTHEWS, W.S. and BARABAS, G. (1981) Suicide and epilepsy: a review of the literature. *Psychosomatics*, 22, 515–524.

MEIER, M.J. and FRENCH, L.A. (1965) Some personality correlates of unilateral and bilateral EEG abnormalities in psychomotor epilepsy. *J. Clin. Psychol.*, 21, 3–9.

MENDEZ, M.F., CUMMINGS, J.L. and BENSON, D.F. (1986) Depression in epilepsy. *Arch. Neurol.*, 43, 766–770.

MELLOR, D.H., LOWIT, I. and HALL, D.J. (1974) Are epileptic children behaviourally different from other children? In *Epilepsy – Proceedings of the Hans Berger Centenary Symposium*, pp. 313–316 (eds. P. HARRIS and C. MAWDSLEY). Churchill Livingstone, Edinburgh.

MIGNONE, R.J., DONNELLY, E.G. and SADOWSKY, D. (1970) Psychological and neurological comparisons of psychomotor and non-psychomotor epileptic patients. *Epilepsia*, 11, 345–359.

MODLIN, H.C. (1960) A study of the MMPI in clinical practice. In *Basic Readings on the MMPI in Psychology and Medicine*, pp. 388–402 (eds G.S. WELSH and W.G. DAHLSTROM), University of Minnesota Press, Minneapolis.

MULDER, D.W. and DALY, D. (1952) Psychiatric symptoms associated with lesions of the temporal lobe. *JAMA*, 150, 173–176.

NIELSEN, H. and KRISTENSEN, O. (1981) Personality correlates of sphenoidal EEG-foci in temporal lobe epilepsy. *Acta. Neurol. Scand.*, 64, 289–300.

OJEMANN, L.M., FRIEL, P.N., TREJO, W.J. and DUDLEY, D.L. (1983) Effect of doxepin on seizure frequency in depressed epileptic patients. *Neurology*, 33, 646–648.

OKUMA, T., INANAGA, K., OTSUKI, S., SARAI, K., TAKAHASHI R., HAZAMA, H., MORI, A. and WATANABE, M. (1981) A preliminary double-blind study of the efficacy of carbamazepine in prophylaxis of manic depressive illness. *Psychopharmacology*, **73**, 95–96.

PALIA, S.S. and HARPER, M.A. (1986) Mood disorders in epilepsy: a survey of psychiatric patients. Presented at the Annual Meeting of the Royal College of Psychiatrists, The University of Southampton, 8–10 July.

PAZZANGIA, P. and FRANK-PAZZANGIA, L. (1976) Record in grade school of pupils with epilepsy: an epidemiological study. *Epilepsia*, **17**, 361–366.

PERINI, G. and MENDIUS, R. (1984) Depression and anxiety in complex partial seizures. *J. Nerv. Ment. Dis.*, **172**, 287–290.

PERINI, G. SUNY, M.D. and MENDIUS, R. (1983) Interictal emotions and behavioural profiles in left and right temporal lobe epileptics. *Psychomatic Med.*, **45**, 83.

POST, R.M., UHDE, T.W., JOFFE, R.T., ROY-BYRNE, P.P. and KELLNER, C. (1985) Anticonvulsant drugs in psychiatric illness: new treatment alternatives and theoretical implications. In *Psychopharmacology of Epilepsy*, pp. 141–171 (ed. M.R. TRIMBLE), John Wiley & Sons, Chichester.

REYNOLDS, J.R. (1861) *Epilepsy: its Symptoms, Treatment and Relation to the Chronic Convulsive Diseases*. Churchill, London.

ROBERTS, J.K.A., ROBERTSON, M.M. and TRIMBLE, M.R. (1982) The lateralising significance of hypergraphia in temporal lobe epilepsy. *J. Neurol. Neurosurg. Psychiatry*, **45**, 131–138.

ROBERTSON, M.M. (1986) Ictal and interictal depression in patients with epilepsy. In *Aspects of Epilepsy and Psychiatry*, pp. 213–234 (eds M.R. TRIMBLE and T.G. BOLWIG), John Wiley & Sons, Chichester.

ROBERTSON, M.M. and TRIMBLE, M.R. (1985) The treatment of depression in patients with epilepsy: a double-blind trial. *J. Affective Disorders*, **9**, 127–136.

ROBERTSON, M.M., TRIMBLE, M.R. and TOWNSEND, H.R.A. (1987) The phenomenology of depression in epilepsy. *Epilepsia*, **28(4)**, 364–372.

RODIN, E. and SCHMALTZ, S. (1984) The Bear–Fedio Personality Inventory and temporal lobe epilepsy. *Neurology*, **34**, 591–596.

RODIN, E.A., KATZ, M. and LENNOX, K. (1976) Differences between patients with temporal lobe seizures and those with other forms of epileptic attacks. *Epilepsia*, **17**, 313–320.

ROY, A. (1979) Some determinants of affective symptoms in epileptics. *Can. J. Psych.*, **24**, 554–556.

SCHOFIELD, A. and DUANE, A. (1986) Organic pathology and psychiatric morbidity in neurological referrals to a consultation/liaison service. Presented at the Royal College of Psychiatrists Annual Meeting, 8–10 July, Southampton.

SERAFETINIDES, E.A. (1975) Psychosocial aspects of neurosurgical management of epilepsy. In *Advances in Neurology*, **8**, p. 323, (eds D.P. PURPURA and U.K. PENRY), Raven Press, New York.

STANDAGE, K.F. and FENTON, G.W. (1975) Psychiatric symptom profiles of patients with epilepsy: a controlled investigation. *Psychol. Med.*, **5**, 152–160.

STEVENS, J.R. (1975) Interictal clinical manifestations of complex partial seizures. In *Advances in Neurology*, (eds J.K. PENRY and D.D. DALY), Raven Press, New York.

TAYLOR, D.C. (1972) Mental state and temporal lobe epilepsy: a correlative account of 100 patients treated surgically. *Epilepsia*, **13**, 727–765.

THOMPSON, P.J. and TRIMBLE, M.R. (1982) Anticonvulsant drugs and cognitive functions. *Epilepsia*, **23**, 531–544.

TOONE, B.J., GARRALDA, M.F. and RON, M.A. (1982) The psychoses of epilepsy and the functional psychoses: a clinical and phenomenological comparison. *Br. J. Psychiat.*, **141**, 256–261.

TOONE, B.K. and DRIVER, N.V. (1980) Psychosis and epilepsy. *Research and Clinical Forums*, **2**, 121–127.

TRIMBLE, M.R. (1978) Non-monoamine oxidase inhibitor antidepressants and epilepsy: a review. *Epilepsia*, **19**, 241–250.

TRIMBLE, M.R. and PEREZ, M. (1982a) Quantification of psychopathology in adult patients with epilepsy. In *Epilepsy and Behaviour '79* and Proceedings of WOPSASSEPY I 1980, pp. 118–126 (eds B.M. KULIG, H. MEINARDI and G. STORES), Swets and Zeitlinger, Lisse.

TRIMBLE, M.R. and PEREZ, M. (1982b) The phenomenology of the chronic psychoses of epilepsy. *Adv. Biol. Psychiat.*, **8**, 98–105.

TRIMBLE, M.R. and ROBERTSON, M.M. (1987) Laterality and psychopathology: recent findings in epilepsy. In *Laterality and Psychopathology*, **3**, pp. 359–369 (eds P. FLOR-HENRY and J. GRUZELIER), Elsevier, North-Holland.

TRIMBLE, M.R., ANLEZARK, G. and MELDRUM, B. (1977) Seizure activity in photosensitive baboons following antidepressant drugs and the role of serotoninergic mechanisms. *Psychopharmacology*, **51**, 159–164.

TUCKER, W.M. and FORSTER, F.M. (1950) Petit mal epilepsy occurring in status. *Arch. Neurol. Psych.*, **64**, 823–827.

WANNEMAKER, B.B. (1983) Unexplained mortality in epilepsy: a perspective on death of patients with epilepsy. Presented at the 15th Epilepsy International Symposium, Washington DC.

WEIL, A.A. (1955) Depressive reactions associated with temporal lobe-uncinate seizures. *J. Nerv. Ment. Dis.*, **121**, 505–510.

WEIL, A.A. (1959) Ictal emotions occurring in temporal lobe dysfunction. *Arch. Neurol.*, **1**, 87–97.

WEISSMAN, M.N. (1981) Antidepressants and psychotherapy in depression. *Adv. Biol. Psych.*, **7**, 230–239.

WELLS, C.E. (1975) Transient ictal psychosis. *Arch. Gen. Psych.*, **32**, 1201–1203.

WHITE, E.W. (1900) Epilepsy associated with insanity. *J. Ment. Sci.*, **46**, 73–79.

WHITMAN, S., HERMANN, B.P. and GORDON, A.C. (1984) Psychopathology in epilepsy: how great is the risk? *Biol. Psych.*, **19(2)**, 213–236.

WILLIAMS, D. (1956) The structure of emotions reflected in epileptic experiences. *Brain*, **79**, 29–67.

WOLF, P. (1982) Manic episodes in epilepsy. In *Advances in Epileptology*, 13th Epilepsy International Symposium, pp. 237–240 (eds H. AKIMOTO, H. KAZAMATSURI, M. SEINO and A.A. WARD), Raven Press, New York.

Discussion

Section IV

Dr J. Moran (Galway): Dr Trimble, in view of the very serious adverse effects found with phenytoin in volunteers and people with epilepsy, could you give us your views on phenytoin in therapeutics?

Dr M.R. Trimble: I rarely use it, unless I am forced to. The anti-epileptic efficacy of the major anticonvulsants is very similar, with the exception of the superiority of carbamazepine for partial complex seizures reported by Dr Smith (p. 83). So choice depends on which drug has the better profile of side-effects. I see a lot of people who have behavioural disturbances associated with epilepsy, and carbamazepine is the drug of choice since its behavioural toxicity profile is the best. The number of new patients who are still put on phenytoin surprises me, especially young girls. The psychosocial consequences of the somatic changes which occur with that drug are often not taken into account, and neither is the teratogenic potential. Further, its pharmokinetics make it difficult to handle, especially in a non-compliant patient.

Professor J.A. Corbett: Would anyone care to comment on the role of folic acid in cognitive deterioration and mood disorders?

Dr M.R. Trimble: Serum or red cell folate deficiency has been associated with poor cognitive performance, psychoses and affective disorder in patients with epilepsy in several studies. These include my own on children at Lingfield Hospital School, and one in association with Dr Robertson on affective disorder in adults. Low folate is also associated with polytherapy, and the prescription of barbituates and phenytoin. Folate plays an essential role in the CNS in several metabolic processes, and it is unlikely that these findings are due to chance.

Dr M.M. Robertson: There are at least five studies in people with epilepsy that show significantly lower serum and red blood folic acid in association either with behaviour disorder in children or affective disorder in adults.

Professor J.A. Corbett: I only know of one study in children giving folic acid in the case of behavioural disorders, which was ineffective. Has it been used in treatment?

159

Dr E.H. Reynolds: There have been positive studies from Botez in Canada and Carney in England in depressed patients. They were not epileptic.

Professor J.A. Corbett: What is significant is that there have been so few studies.

Dr E.H. Reynolds: There have been negative trials of folic acid in epileptic patients, many years ago.

Professor N. O'Donohoe (Dublin): Dr Smith suggested that primidone was a far better tolerated drug than phenobarbitone. In paediatrics for many years primidone and phenobarbitone have been tarred with the same brush. They are both disadvantageous for children, and pharmacologists have told us that perhaps they work identically. I would like to have his comments on primidone versus phenobarbitone.

Dr D.B. Smith: Nearly one third of the patients taking primidone in our study dropped out within the first month because of intolerable toxicity. The toxicity was primarily systemic; it was nausea, vomiting and dizziness. We were left with a highly selected group who tolerated primidone. However, those patients did extremely well. It is different from phenobarbitone. It does have some positive psychotropic effects, and it did not result in the same degree of deterioration on many of the sub-tests of the behavioural toxicity battery that we found with phenobarbitone. However the phenobarbitone levels were considerably lower in the patients on primidone. They ranged anywhere from 8 to 14 micrograms/ml as opposed to average levels in the phenobarbitone patients of 23 micrograms/ml. The degree of seizure control in patients on primidone was equal to that of phenobarbitone, so anti-epileptic effects of primidone itself are important. I think that primidone is a different drug and if tolerated has advantages in terms of its neuropsychological effects.

Question from the floor: Is there any specific cognitive or behavioural pattern or subset which indicates a drug effect?

Dr P.J. Thompson: There are certain indicators, like slowing, which relate to drugs.

Dr M.R. Trimble: Slowing is one of the crucial variables, but a number of neurological processes can cause slowing; you see it in multiple sclerosis and Parkinson's disease for example.

Question from the floor: So there are certain patterns which make you suspect a drug effect?

Dr M.R. Trimble: I can go one step further, with a personal anecdote. A girl who had Sturge-Weber syndrome, who was intellectually retarded, was virtually moribund at home. She was doubly incontinent, very apathetic and lethargic and needed full-time attention from her mother. She came to me on phenytoin monotherapy (300 mgms a day), serum levels within the therapeutic range, which she had been on for two or three years; before that she had been on polytherapy. I changed her to carbamazepine monotherapy and six months later she was in a day centre, no longer doubly incontinent, making friends, etc. Her mother no longer had to look after her all the time.

Dr E.H. Reynolds: Drugs specifically affect drive, initiative, mood, arousal, and sociability.

Dr M.R. Trimble: We get a number of patients referred to us as 'depressed' but actually they are not, they are dysphoric and they are suffering from effects of polytherapy.

Dr D. Mellor (Nottingham): Some patients seem to be a lot better in themselves after having a few fits. The usual analogy is with ECT. Have you looked at the fluctuation of the level of depression with the seizure frequency?

Dr M.M. Robertson: In the literature there are some studies that found seizure frequency to be less prior to the onset of a depressive illness. However, documentation of out-patient seizure frequency begs questions at the best of times, especially if the patient is becoming depressed.

Dr M. Harper (Cardiff): Can I pursue that a little further. I'm sure we have all had patients who have either developed a psychosis or severe depression when their fits are controlled in the absence of evident drug toxicity. Does Landolt's concept of forced normalization help us?

Dr M.R. Trimble: It was a purely descriptive term. In English the term 'forced normalization' implies some mechanism, but Landolt apparently used it descriptively. Tellenbach introduced the concept of alternating psychosis, which is probably better from the point of view of clinicians since it does not rely on the EEG phenomenon but on the clinical pattern. These are patients who, when their seizures come under control develop a psychosis and vice versa. Wolf has made the point that it is not only psychosis that needs to be considered but also other behaviours. Paediatricians are familiar with the fact that occasionally you get a child's seizures under control but their behaviour deteriorates. They are not psychotic but they develop a conduct disorder. As Tellenbach pointed out, these cases are important from the point of view of epilepsy because you have the choice of taking away the seizures and producing a behaviour problem or letting the patient have seizures. Treating the seizures is not treating the patient.

Dr E.H. Reynolds: Many things relate to this issue. For example, catatonic schizophrenics may develop seizures spontaneously. Denis Hill viewed this as a homeostatic mechanism in schizophrenia. Phenothiazines are epileptogenic in schizophrenics. There are other observations relating to methionine, methionine sulfoxamine, folic acid and monoamines.

Dr D.B. Smith: Anti-epileptic drugs may cause some depression.

Dr M.R. Trimble: I do not think it is all drugs. There is another setting where you see this same phenomenon, that is after temporal lobectomy. We have seen several patients, dramatically relieved of seizures, that develop an acute post-operature affective psychosis. Further, you treat depressive illness with a seizure when you give people ECT.

Dr J. Green (Manchester): The same phenomenon is seen the other way round in a prodrome to a seizure. Certainly in children, you see a gradual rise in temperature in terms of behaviour, general arousal and dysthymia which is resolved after the fit. This is fairly common.

Section V

12

Memory and epilepsy

PIERRE LOISEAU*, EVELYN STRUBE* and JEAN-LOUIS SIGNORET†
*Hôpital Pellegrin, Université de Bordeaux II, France and †Hôpital de la
Salpêtrière, Université de Paris VI, France

INTRODUCTION

It is difficult and to some extent inadequate to consider memory apart from
other neuropsychological functions (Reitan, 1977). Even so, memory deficits
in epileptic patients merit special attention since they seek help for these more
frequently than for other mental impairments.

Interest in this area is not new. In his *Traité de l'Epilepsie*, Tissot (1770)
wrote that he had never seen an epileptic whose fits were not very rare not
complaining about a weakening of memory. And a century later, Gowers
(1881) wrote: 'The mental state of epileptics, as is well known, frequently
presents deterioration . . . In its slighter form there is merely defective memory, especially for recent acquisitions.' But all epileptic patients do not
deteriorate nor have defective memories. Considering the mental condition of
epileptics during the intervals between attacks, Reynolds (1861) concluded
that epilepsy does not necessarily involve any mental change, but 'it appears
that it is more common to find a defective than a normal memory. Further,
when memory is defective, its most frequent condition is that of slight but
general impairment.'

A substantial body of literature on neuropsychological functioning in
epilepsy is now available. However, some lack of agreement still persists. The
importance and even the existence of a memory loss are disputed (Scott et al.,
1967). The parts of the memory processes impaired by epilepsy are not well
defined. None the less, studies carried out to investigate memory in epileptic
patients generally confirm the clinicians' opinion that, for memory tasks, the
performance levels of these patients are lower than those of healthy subjects.

What are the reasons for and the nature of these memory impairments? Partial answers now exist for these two questions.

FACTORS INFLUENCING MEMORY DISORDERS IN EPILEPSY

A number of factors influence the memory disturbances in epileptic patients. However their importance has been diversely appreciated. For instance, Reynolds (1861) wrote that the more frequent the seizures, the more pronounced the memory troubles, but that the age at onset of the disease and its duration were of no importance. Gowers claimed just the contrary.

The main factors are as follows.

Presence of brain damage

The performance of brain-damaged epileptic patients is lower than that of patients with epilepsy of unknown origin (Matthews and Kløve, 1967). The presence of the brain damage alone might be responsible for impaired memory functioning. However, it was shown that after a head trauma, seizures increased the impairment (Dikmen and Reitan, 1978).

Frequency of seizures

A greater impairment was associated with a higher seizure frequency for Dikmen and Matthews (1977) but not for Delaney et al. (1980). It is likely that the frequency of seizures does play a role, both directly and indirectly. Directly, because seizures with loss of consciousness disturb mental functioning, not only during the seizure but also afterwards, sometimes for several days. When a test is carried out after a seizure, the score is lower than when obtained far from it: and when seizures are frequent, far is never far. The responsibility of seizures may also be indirect. An ongoing process may occur in chronic epilepsy because of cerebral damage due to repeated seizures (Reynolds et al., 1983). This opinion is supported by recent biochemical studies showing an excess of excitotoxins, such as quinolinic acid, in epileptic foci (Feldblum et al., in press). Mouritzen Dam (1980) demonstrated a relation between the number of seizures and a cell loss in the hippocampus, an essential structure in some memory processes.

Memory functioning as well as other performances can be disturbed by the repetition of not only clinical seizures, but also subictal discharges (Binnie, Chapter 4). Decreased performances are correlated with increasing discharge rates, or length of the discharges, and generalized discharges are worse than focal discharges (Mirsky et al., 1960; Wilkus and Dodrill, 1976; Dodrill, 1980). Glowinski (1973) considered that subictal electrical discharges in temporal lobes disturb memory functioning by directly interrupting memory storage.

Duration of epilepsy

A long duration of epilepsy impairs memory functioning (Mirsky et al., 1960; Ladavas et al., 1979; Delaney et al., 1980). Ten years appears to be a crucial length. In fact, a long duration generally means seizures repeated during many years, and a prolonged therapy. So neither the duration nor the frequency is an independent variable.

Age at onset

An early onset, even if nonsignificant for Delaney et al. (1980), is a recognized deleterious factor (Dikmen et al., 1974; O'Leary et al., 1981).

This, too, overlaps the other ones. Besides, childhood is a very important period for learning, a period during which one learns how to learn.

The electro-clinical form of epilepsy

Considerable evidence has confirmed a complementary specialization of the temporal lobes for information processing and retention in man.

Damage to the left temporal lobe impairs verbal abilities, whereas lesions in the right hemisphere decrease nonverbal, perceptual memory (Piercy, 1964). These findings have been corroborated with subjects who underwent a unilateral temporal lobe resection for intractable seizures (Milner, 1975). However, these findings do not clearly answer the question as to whether nonsurgical epileptic patients have such a specific pattern of deficit. A cortical resection may impair higher functions more than an epileptic focus without a gross anatomical lesion. In monkeys, the ablation of some cortical areas impairs memory much more than focal epileptic discharges (Stamm and Pribram, 1960, 1961). Research with nonsurgical patients has not consistently demonstrated selective memory deficits in temporal lobe epilepsies (Hermann et al., 1987). The discrepancies are probably due to the use of different memory tasks. A specific memory impairment was found in children with temporal-lobe epilepsy, contrasting with normal memory functioning in centrencephalic epilepsy. Children with left temporal epilepsy performed worse than children with right temporal epilepsy (Fedio and Mirsky, 1969). A difference between left and right temporal epilepsy was found only for long-term memory (Ladavas et al., 1979). Delaney et al. (1980) found an impairment of verbal memory tasks in left, and of nonverbal, visual memory tasks in right temporal epilepsy. Hermann et al. (1987) demonstrated that left-temporal epileptic patients had poorer verbal learning ability, impaired immediate memory, an increased difficulty in the retrieval of verbal material and a poor semantic organization in their verbal learning and recall, whereas right temporal patients performed nearly as well as normal controls. Temporal-lobe epileptics have poorer performances than centrencephalic patients who in turn perform less well than controls, but no significant relation was found between the laterality of the temporal epileptogenic lesion and an impairment of verbal and nonverbal memory-task performances on using the Wechsler Memory Scale (Glowinski, 1973).

Anticonvulsant drugs

The influence of anticonvulsant drugs on cognitive functions and, among them, on memory, has recently received much attention (see Trimble and Reynolds, 1976; Thompson and Trimble, 1982; Trimble, 1987).

Detrimental effects of sedative anti-epileptic drugs on memory functioning are well documented (and the main anti-epileptic drugs are sedative) even if existing reports have sometimes been conflicting. A relationship between drug dosage and memory scores has been shown (Reynolds and Travers, 1974). Performance improves after a reduction of dose (Dekaban and Lehman, 1975; Oxley et al., 1979; Thompson and Trimble, 1982). Patients with toxic levels perform worse than patients with non-toxic levels (Matthews and Harley, 1975). More sophisticated data were given by Trimble and Thompson (see Trimble, 1987).

Phenobarbital, phenytoin and primidone intake is clearly an important factor responsible for memory impairment in epileptic patients. Benzodiazepines appear to affect mainly the consolidation of information. Sodium valproate and carbamazepine are certainly less toxic (Dodrill and Troupin, 1977).

However, anti-epileptic drugs cannot entirely account for the defect in memory noted in epileptic patients. With a selected battery of neuropsychological tests, untreated patients scored significantly and consistently below the level of the control subjects (Smith et al., 1985; Chapter 6).

Other factors

A patient's emotional state or motivations may alter memory performance (Lishman, 1972; Hirtz and Nelson, 1985).

In summary, several factors may explain these disturbances of memory. It is obvious that they may often operate in combination. For instance, many seizures are experienced and polypharmacy is taken for years in a difficult-to-treat adult patient in whom fits began during childhood. This patient may have a poor occupational adjustment resulting in a depressive mood.

NATURE OF THE MEMORY IMPAIRMENTS

Overview of the problem

Memory-task deficits have often been demonstrated in selected groups of patients with epilepsy. Some years ago (Loiseau et al., 1983), we addressed the question of memory functioning in epileptic patients encountered in current neurological practice. Two hundred adults with a normal socio-professional adjustment and with no defined cerebral lesion were tested. The test battery was elementary: two subtests of the Wechsler Memory Scale (digits span and geometric figures) for the initial registration and a list of 15 words (Rey, 1970) for recall and recognition.

Our patients performed more poorly than controls matched for age and educational level. In these patients short memory was more impaired than learning, in contrast to the results of Fedio and Mirsky (1979) and Ladavas et al. (1979) in temporal lobe epilepsy. Furthermore, differences were noted according to the educational levels. For example, university-educated patients had an immediate recall superior to that of manual workers, but, on the other hand, the learning scores of these two groups were similar. Such a correlation with education was noted by Smith et al. (1986). Incidentally, neither type of epilepsy, frequency of seizures, duration of illness, nor medication, if considered alone, accounted for this impairment.

The choice of memory tests – influence on results

Our first data were unsatisfactory because the tests were too simple. A similar remark applies to many of the published studies. When cognitive skills are tested with a complete neuropsychological inventory, such as the Halstead–Reitan battery, few items explore memory functioning. The Wechsler Memory Scale, especially when only the Memory Quotient is used, is not discriminative enough. For instance, its subtest 7 failed to demonstrate the well-documented effect of phenytoin. In a recent study (Loiseau et al., in press), 10 out of 11 patients scored normally on two subtests of the Wechsler Memory Scale, whereas they achieved poor performance with another battery. Using insufficiently difficult tasks probably explains why some authors did not find any disturbance of memory in epileptic patients.

We therefore chose Signoret's Memory Battery Scale (Signoret and Whiteley, 1979). This battery permits quantification of memory functioning in discrete situations. For each situation, verbal and visual material of similar difficulty is used. The scores are for: (1) immediate recall of a structural entity, either verbal (logical story), or visual (a complex geometric figure); (2) immediate free recall of a list of unrelated words or series of geometrical figures with three learning trials; (3) delayed recall of the structural entity; (4) delayed recall of the words and of the figures; (5) recognition of previously learned items mixed with new items; (6) learning of five associated pairs with three trials. This allows the investigation of initial registration, learning (retrieval and recognition) and forgetfulness.

In 1982 this battery was presented to 56 adults with the same characteristics as in our first study. It confirmed our previous results with more details. Patient scores were significantly worse than those of matched controls; no difference was observed between generalized and partial epilepsy; the length of illness and the frequency of seizures were consistently correlated with poor memory abilities; the impairment was obviously multifactorial. More interesting, poor memory performance was mainly due to a recall deficiency. We concluded that epileptic patients have difficulties in learning but remember well what they have learned.

We recently studied a rather homogeneous group of 27 patients. They were adult, had frequent complex partial seizures (26 of them had more than four seizures per month) and were in the difficult-to-treat category. A control group consisted of normal subjects, matched for sex, age and years of schooling. The main results were as follows (see also Table 1):

1. As a group, the epileptic patients scored significantly lower than the controls ($p < 0.01$ to $p < 0.0001$) except in one task (verbal recognition).
2. The initial registration was impaired, for the short story as well as for the complex figure ($p < 0.001$).
3. The immediate recall of a list of words was relatively less impaired after three presentations ($p < 0.01$), but was very low after the first presentation ($p < 0.001$). This was in keeping with previous analyses of memory loss in temporal lobe epilepsy. Patients with the opportunity to practise improved on a word task, but their performance dropped when the task was timed

Table 1.   Signoret memory battery scale: p value patients/controls

	Epileptic Pts (N = 27)	Vascular Pts (N = 11)	Head trauma Pts (N = 21)
Verbal			
Immediate recall (story)	<.001	n.s.	<.0001
Immediate recall (words)	<.01	n.s.	<.001
Delayed recall (story)	<.0001	n.s.	<.0001
Delayed recall (words)	<.01	n.s.	<.001
Recognition	n.s.	n.s.	<.01
Associated learning	<.001	n.s.	<.01
Visual			
Immediate recall (figure)	<.001	n.s.	<.0001
Immediate recall (figures)	<.0001	<.05	<.0001
Delayed recall (figure)	<.001	n.s.	<.001
Delayed recall (figures)	<.001	n.s.	<.0001
Recognition	<.002	n.s.	n.s.
Associated learning	<.001	n.s.	<.001

(Berent et al., 1980). The hypothesis most frequently used to explain the memory deficit in epileptic patients has been that it involves the consolidation of the memory trace or the transfer of the memory trace from short-term memory to long-term storage. A lesion of either temporal lobe decreases auditory-processing capabilities thus inducing a reduction in coding (Delaney et al., 1982). We believe, however, that this difficulty is not limited to patients with a temporal-lobe epilepsy. The initial encoding of information may also be impaired by the slowness of many patients. This slowness may be drug-induced. Patients tested prior to and after initiation of drug therapy have a normal digit span before the administration of antiepileptic drugs, and a decreased digit span when under medication (Smith et al., 1980). More frequent and longer presentations of the material improve the memory scores (Stores, 1981).

It appears that the learning difficulty in epileptic patients is, at least partly, due to a poor initial encoding of information. The impairment of delayed recall is its consequence. This could explain why the delayed recall of the story was clearly inferior (p<0.0001) to that of the list of words (p<0.01) which benefited from three learning trials.

4. The results with the visual tasks did not demonstrate such a difference. According to Pavio's dual theory (Horton and Bergfeld Mills, 1984), in normal subjects, pictures are stored in both a verbal- and an image-memory system, and hence are remembered better. A decreased or slowed verbal encoding in epileptic patients could explain their poor performance on visual tasks, especially when a series of meangingless figures has to be learned (p<0.0001). Patients as well as controls explained that for remembering the figures they put a name on them: a snail, a worm, etc.

5. When individual patients' scores were compared to the mean of the controls' scores, five out of 27 patients had a normal performance. All the epileptics do not have a memory impairment.

6. We did not find any significant difference between patients with a unilateral left or right temporal focus for verbal or non-verbal memory tasks. The lack of clear influence of lateralization in some epileptic patients could be explained by the nature of the epileptogenic focus. The presence of a lesion influences the interhemispheric pattern in perceptual and attentional tasks: it shifts the prevalence to the hemisphere without a lesion (Mazzuchi et al., 1985). A lesion of either hemisphere appears capable of interfering with language and verbal-memory functioning in a high proportion of patients (Powell et al., 1987). Electroclinical signs as they are usually obtained are probably insufficient for determining the lateralization of functions in these patients. However, efforts to assess the functional role of each temporal lobe are worthwhile (Hermann et al., 1987). Neuro-imaging could provide substantial information on the part(s) of the brain involved in verbal and visual tasks.

Memory and attention

The ability to maintain attention is necessary for the initial registration of verbal and visual material. An impairment of attention was demonstrated in patients with a so-called centrencephalic epilepsy (Mirsky et al., 1960; Lansdell and Mirsky, 1964; Fedio and Mirsky, 1969). However, a distracting task caused decreased memory performance for both temporal and centrencephalic patients (Glowinski, 1973). Epileptic children perform attention tasks poorly (Stores et al., 1978). Anticonvulsant drugs are known to affect attention (Dekaban and Lehman, 1975; Matthews and Harley, 1975; Trimble 1987).

A variety of attentional tasks have been used. The aim of one of our studies (Loiseau et al., 1984) was to look for a correlation between attention and memory in epileptic patients. Epileptic patients were significantly inferior to controls ($p < 0.001$) but, in contrast to the Mirsky group results, the impairment was more marked for partial than for generalized epilepsies. We used a new Attentional Battery. A further comparison between this battery designed for brain-damaged patients and other attentional tasks, cast a doubt on its sensitivity in epilepsy. We now use (1) a code test (measure of speed: the subject must write on one side of a file of letters a corresponding figure; (2) the Zazzo test (measure of a choice: the subject must cross out one type or two types of tailed squares among other tailed squares; (3) the Stroop test (decision-making and flexibility: in a modified form of the classical Stroop procedure (Dodrill, 1978) the subject must read the words down the page, regardless of their colour, and then state the colour of ink, ignoring the words). In the above-mentioned group of difficult-to-treat patients we confirmed low-attentional performances (Table 2).

We addressed the question of the role of clearly unilateral lesions in attentional and memory performances. Non-aphasic cerebro-vascular patients were examined. Elderly patients were excluded. These patients performed more poorly than their controls ($p < 0.05$ to 0.001) on attentional tasks (Table 2), but did not significantly differ from controls on memory tasks (Table 1).

Table 2.   Attention tasks

	Epileptic Pts (N = 27)	Vascular Pts (N = 11)	Head trauma Pts (N = 21)
Zazzo test (one sign)	<.001	<.01	<.0001
Zazzo test (two signs)	<.001	<.01	<.0001
Stroop test (words)	<.0001	<.05	<.001
Stroop test (colours)	<.0001	<.001	<.0001
Code	<.0001	<.001	<.0001

Our conclusion is that decreased attention is probably insufficient to explain memory disability.

Lastly, a group of patients having had a severe head trauma was investigated with the same attentional and memory tasks. They had diffuse cerebral lesions. The presence of cognitive defects following head injury is clearly established (Brooks, 1983). Memory and attention are particularly vulnerable (Levin et al., 1982). These patients were markedly inferior to controls for both memory and attentional tasks (Tables 1 and 2). The deficit was severer than in epileptic patients. This suggests an important role for diffuse cerebral lesions in memory and attention.

CONCLUSION

Memory skills are decreased in many epileptic patients, but not in all patients, because of a primary disturbance of amnestic processes and because of decreased attention. Bilateral lesions are probably necessary. These lesions can be either structural or functional, resulting from repeated seizures and/or from anti-epileptic drugs.

The lack of agreement in the literature calls for further studies (i) taking into account the factors which may operate often in combination; and (ii) using very sensitive measures of memory.

ACKNOWLEDGEMENTS

The authors would like to thank Edwidge Richer MD, and Xavier Debelleix MD, for the opportunity to study their patients. They would like to acknowledge the assistance of Edith Magnen in testing the patients and providing controls, of Jim Sneed for help in preparing the manuscript and Marie-Francoise Aury for typing and processing this manuscript.

REFERENCES

BERENT, S., BOLL, T.J. and GIORDANI, B. (1980) Hemispheric site of epileptogenic focus: cognitive, perceptual, and psychosocial implications for children and adults. In *Advances in Epileptology*, XIth Epilepsy International Symposium (eds R. CANGER, F. ANGELERI and J.K. PENRY), pp. 185–190. Raven Press, New York.

BROOKS, D.N. (1983) Cognitive deficits after head injury. In *Closed Head Injury* (eds D.N. BROOKS). Oxford University Press, Oxford.

DEKABAN, A.S. and LEHMAN, E.J.B. (1975) Effects of different dosages of anticonvulsant drugs on mental performance in patients with chronic epilepsy. *Acta Neurol. Scand.*, 52, 319–330.

DELANEY, R.C., ROSEN, A.J., MATTSON, R.H. and NOVELLY, R.A. (1980) Memory function in focal epilepsy: a comparison of non surgical, unilateral temporal lobe and frontal lobe samples. *Cortex*, 16, 103–117.

DELANEY, R.C., PREVEY, M.L. and MATTSON, R.H. (1982) Short term retention with lateralized temporal lobe epilepsy. *Cortex*, **22**, 591–600.

DIKMEN, S. and MATTHEWS, C.G. (1977) Effect of major motor seizure frequency upon cognitive-intellectual functions in adults. *Epilepsia*, **18**, 21–29.

DIKMEN, S. and REITAN, R.M. (1978). Neuropsychological performance in post-traumatic epilepsy. *Epilepsia*, **19**, 177–183.

DIKMEN, S., MATTHEWS, C.G. and HARLEY, J.P. (1975) The effect of early versus late onset of major motor epilepsy upon cognitive-intellectual performance. *Epilepsia*, **16**, 73–81.

DODRILL, C.B. (1978) A neuropsychological battery for epilepsy. *Epilepsia*, **19**, 611–623.

DODRILL, C.B. (1980) Neuropsychological evaluation in epilepsy. In *Epilepsy: A Window to Brain Mechanisms* (eds J.S. LOCKARD and A.A. WARD Jr), pp. 231–241. Raven Press, New York.

DODRILL, C.B. and TROUPIN, A.S. (1977). Psychotropic effects of carbamazepine in epilepsy. A double-blind comparison with phenytoin. *Neurology*, **27**, 1023–1028.

FEDIO, P. and MIRSKY, A.F. (1969) Selective intellectual deficits in children with temporal lobe or centrencephalic epilepsy. *Neuropsychologia*, **7**, 287–300.

FELDBLUM, S., ROUGIER, A., LOISEAU, H., LOISEAU, P., COHADON, F., MORSELLI, P.L. and LLOYD, K.G. Quinolinic-phosphoribosyltransferase is decreased in epileptic human brain tissue, *Epilepsia* (in press).

GLOWINSKI, H. (1973) Cognitive deficits in temporal lobe epilepsy. An investigation of memory functioning. *J. Nerv. Ment. Dis.*, **157**, 129–137.

GOWERS, W.R. (1881) *Epilepsy and Other Chronic Convulsive Diseases: their causes, symptoms and treatment*, Churchill, London.

HERMANN, B.P., WYLER, A.R., RICHEY, E.T. and REA, J.M. (1987) Memory function and verbal learning ability in patients with complex partial seizures of temporal lobe origin. *Epilepsia*, **28**, 547–554.

HIRTZ, D.G. and NELSON, K.B. (1985) Cognitive effects of antiepileptic drugs. In *Recent Advances in Epileptology* (ed. B.S. MELDRUM), pp. 161–181, Churchill, Edinburgh.

HORTON, D.L. and BERGFELD MILLS, C. (1984) Human learning and memory. *Ann. Rev. Psychol.*, **35**, 361–394.

LADAVAS, E., UMILTA, C. and PROVINCIALI, L. (1979) Hemisphere-dependent cognitive performances in epileptic patients. *Epilepsia*, **20**, 493–502.

LANSDELL, H. and MIRSKY, A.F. (1964) Attention in focal and centrencephalic epilepsy. *Exp. Neurol*, **9**, 463–465.

LEVIN, H., BENTON, A. and GROSSMAN, R. (1982) *Behavioral Consequences of Closed Head Injury*. Oxford University Press, New York.

LISHMAN, W.A. (1972) Selective factors in memory: Part 2: Affective disorder. *Psychol. Med.*, **2**, 248–253.

LOISEAU, P., SIGNORET, J.L., STRUBE, E., BROUSTET, D. and DARTIGUES, J.F. (1982). Nouveaux procédés d'appréciation des troubles de la mémoire chez les epileptiques. *Rev. Neurol.* (Paris), **138**, 387–400.

LOISEAU, P., STRUBE, E., BROUSTET, D., BATTELLOCHI, S., GOMENI, C. and MORSELLI, P.L. (1983) Learning impairment in epileptic patients. *Epilepsia*, **24**, 183–192.

LOISEAU, P., SIGNORET, J.L. and STRUBE, E. (1984) Attention problems in adult epileptic patients. *Acta Neurol. Scand.*, **69**, Suppl. **99**, 31–34.

LOISEAU, P., STRUBE, E., TOR, J., LEVY, R.H. and DODRILL, C.B. Evaluation neuro-psychologique et thérapeutique du stiripentol dans l'épilepsie. Résultats prélimi-naires. *Rev. Neurol.* (Paris) (in press).

MATTHEWS, C.G. and HARLEY, J.P. (1975) Differential psychological test performances in toxic and non toxic adult epileptics. *Neurology*, **25**, 184–188.

MATTHEWS, C.G. and KLØVE, H. (1967) Differential psychological performances in major motor, psychomotor and mixed seizures classifications of known and unknown etiology. *Epilepsia*, **8**, 117–128.

MAZZUCCHI, A., VISINTINI, D., MAGNANI, G., CATTELANI, R. and PARMA, M. (1985) Hemispheric prevalence changes in partial epileptic patients on perceptual and attentional tasks. *Epilepsia*, **26**, 379–390.

MILNER, B. (1975) Psychological aspects of focal epilepsy and its neurosurgical management. In *Advances in Neurology*, **8** (eds D.P. PURPURA, J.K. PENRY and R.D. WALKER), pp. 299–321. Raven Press, New York.

MIRSKY, A.F., PRIMAC, D.W., MARSAN, C.A., ROSVOLD, H.E. and STEVENS, J.R. (1960) A comparison of the psychological test performance of patients with focal and non focal epilepsy, *Exp. Neurol.* **2**, 75–89.

MOURITZEN DAM, A. (1980) Epilepsy and neuron loss in the hippocampus. *Epilepsia*, **21**, 617–629.

O'LEARY, D.S., SEIDENBERG, M., BERENT, S. and BOLL, T.J. (1981) Effects of age of onset of tonic-clonic seizures on neuropsychological performance in children. *Epilepsia*, **22**, 197–204.

OXLEY, J., RICHENS, A. and WADSWORTH, J. (1979) Improvement in memory function in epileptic subjects following a reduction in serum phenobarbitone level. In *11th Epilepsy International Symposium* Abstract 226, 30 Sept.–3 Oct. Florence.

PIERCY, M. (1964) The effects of cerebral lesions on intellectual functions; a review of current research trends, *Br. J. Psychiat.*, **110**, 310–352.

POWELL, G.E., POLKEY, C.E. and CANAVAN, A.G.M. (1987) Lateralisation of memory functions in epileptic patients by use of the sodium amytal (Wada) technique. *J. Neurol. Neurosurg. Psychiat.*, **50**, 665–672.

REITAN, R.M. (1977) Psychological testing of epileptic patients. In *The Epilepsies, Handbook of Clinical Neurology*, **15** (eds P.J. VINKEN and G.W. BRUYN), pp. 559–575. Elsevier, Amsterdam.

REY, A. (1970) *Les Troubles de mémoire et leur examen psychométrique*, Dessart, Publ., Paris.

REYNOLDS, E.H. and TRAVERS, R.D. (1974) Serum anticonvulsant concentration in epileptic patients with mental symptoms. *Br. J. Psychiat.*, **124**, 440–445.

REYNOLDS, E.H., ELWES, R.D.C. and SHORVON, S.D. (1983) Why does epilepsy become intractable? Prevention of chronic epilepsy. *Lancet*, **ii**, 952–954.

REYNOLDS, J.R. (1861) *Epilepsy: its symptoms, treatment and relation to other chronic convulsive diseases*. Churchill, London.

SCOTT, D.F., MOFFATT, A., MATTHEWS, A. and ETTLINGER, G. (1967) The effect of epileptic discharges on learning and memory in patients. *Epilepsia*, **8**, 188–194.

SIGNORET, J.L. and WHITELEY, A. (1979) Memory battery scale. *INS Bulletin*, **2**, 26.

SMITH, D.B., CRAFT, B.R., COLLINS, J., MATTSON, R.H. and CRAMER, J.A. (1986) Behavioral characteristics of epileptic patients compared with normal controls, *Epilepsia*, **27**, 760–768.

STAMM, J.S. and PRIBRAM, K.H. (1960) Effects of epileptogenic lesions in frontal cortex on learning and retention in monkeys. *J. Neurophysiol.*, **23**, 552–563.

STAMM, J.S. and PRIBRAM, K.K. (1961) Effects of epileptogenic lesions in inferotemporal cortex on learning and retention in monkey. *J. Comp. Physiol. Psychol.*, **54**, 614–618.

STORES, G. (1981) Memory impairment in children with epilepsy. *Acta Neurol. Scand.*, **64**, suppl. **89**, 21–27.

STORES, G., HART, J. and PIRAN, N. (1978) Inattentiveness in school children with epilepsy. *Epilepsia,* **19**, 169–175.

THOMPSON, P.J. and TRIMBLE, M.R. (1982). Anticonvulsant drugs and cognitive functions. *Epilepsia,* **23**, 531–544.

TISSOT, S.A. (1770) *Traité de l'épilepsie, faisant le tôme troisième de traité des nerfs et de leurs maladies.* Paris.

TRIMBLE, M.R. (1987) Les effets cognitifs des médicaments antiépileptiques, *Rev. Neurol.* (Paris), **143**, 420–428.

TRIMBLE, M.R. and REYNOLDS, E.H. (1976) Anticonvulsant drugs and mental symptoms: a review. *Psychol. Med.,* **6**, 169–178.

WESCHLER, D. (1945) A standardized memory scale for clinical use, *J. Psychol.,* **19**, 87–95.

WILKUS, R.J. and DODRILL, C.B. (1976) Neuropsychological correlates of the electroencephalogram in epileptics. I. Topographic distribution and average rate of epileptiform activity. *Epilepsia,* **17**, 89–100.

13

Dementia in epileptic patients

Stephen W. Brown and Margaret Vaughan
The David Lewis Centre for Epilepsy, Warford, Cheshire

The mind is slowly weakened by the storms of fury through which it passes, and they sink finally into the apathy of dementia – a state of mere oblivion, in which they cease to hope or care more.

Maudsley (1874)

The most numerous class of epileptics show, after the lapse of years, a slowly progressive dimming of the active perceptions of the mind, a loss of memory, a blunting of the affections, a permanent mental obtuseness which increases and grows until, if the patient lives long enough, there is a more or less absolute annihilation of all the faculties.

Berkley (1901)

The mental state of epileptics, as is well known, frequently presents deterioration . . . in the slighter form there is merely a defective memory . . . in more severe degrees there is a greater impairment of mental power, weakened capacity for attention and often defective moral control.

Gowers (1881)

INTRODUCTION

Throughout the nineteenth and early twentieth centuries it was widely accepted that intellectual deterioration was a frequent outcome of epilepsy. Now it is not. Were our Victorian forebears contemplating a different patient group than that which we see today? Has the natural history of seizure disorders mutated in some way with time? Were our predecessors perhaps more observant than us? Or less observant? There is certainly reason to believe that the patient group may have changed; neurosyphilis can cause both seizures and dementia. It was common then and is now rare. This may not be sufficient

177

explanation, however. When psychology came of age as a respectable quantitative science, and the first IQ tests, purporting to measure 'intelligence', were applied to populations of patients with epilepsy, there sometimes was evidence of intellectual deterioration on retesting (Dawson and Conn, 1929). However, it soon became clear that this was part of a phenomenon of fluctuation in test performance which could occur in either direction (Patterson and Fonner, 1928; Fetterman and Barnes, 1934; Sulivan and Gahagan, 1935), and there was a suggestion that improvement in seizure control could enhance IQ test performance (Kugelmass et al., 1938), so that the observed fluctuations on retesting could be related to seizure frequency. Some studies did suggest a slight decline in mean intelligence with increasing duration of seizure disorder, but no very clear picture emerged (Brown and Reynolds, 1982).

Instead, with the development of neuropsychology, the emphasis shifted to identifying discrete cognitive deficits associated with discrete epileptic foci, and since the 1950s a number of interesting studies have examined the relationship of temporal lobe lesions to memory problems (e.g. Delaney et al., 1980; Loisseau, Chapter 12). However no account can be taken in such studies of those patients whose abilities fall outside the standardization range for these neuropsychological tests and who therefore cannot be accurately tested for discrete cognitive deficits. Unfortunately, this would include people with a profound dementia syndrome.

FIRST STUDY

A few years ago (Brown and Abeyasinghe, 1984) we collected a sample of twelve adult patients with epilepsy from the Maudsley and King's College Hospitals who showed evidence for intellectual deterioration based on knowledge of previous educational or vocational attainments which were incompatible with the present level off functioning. This information was supplemented by serial psychometry showing a drop of approximately one standard deviation or more (c.15 points) in Full Scale IQ measured on the Wechsler Adult Intelligence Scale (WAIS), in nine patients. In two patients only a single test result was available, but this was incompatible with previous educational or vocational achievement. In one patient serial psychometry had shown a drop of approximately half a standard deviation (7 points) in Full Scale IQ, but there was evidence of intellectual deterioration before the first IQ test. The mean fall in IQ in the ten patients who had had serial psychometry was 23 points on the verbal IQ (range 8–30), 18 points on Peformance IQ (7–24) and 21.5 points on the Full Scale IQ (7–31). Eight patients were male and four female, and none had a family history of epilepsy. Other seizure variables are shown in Table 1. There was a tendency for patients to have more than one clinical seizure type, as can be seen in Table 2. The seizure total during the year before deterioration was first noted was recovered from case notes. All patients had more than ten

Table 1.   Seizure variables for 12 patients with intellectual deterioration

---

Sex: 8 male 4 female

Mean age onset epilepsy: 10.3 years (range 1–34)

Duration of epilepsy before deterioration noted:
>10 years 7 patients
5–10 years 3 patients
<10 years 2 patients

History of status? 2 patients

Past psychiatric history? 4 patients (2 as inpatients)
1 male = schizoid personality
1 male = postictal psychosis of schizophrenia type
2 females = neurotic problems

Intellectual decline first noted by:
attending physician = 4
patient's family = 4
patient = 3
patient's employer = 1

Symptoms or signs of CNS disease? 4 patients
1 = impaired motor coordination
1 = athetosis of R arm
1 = polyneuropahty
1 = dysarthria

---

seizures in those 12 months and in eight cases more than 50 seizures had occurred. All patients had abnormal EEGs at the time of presentation and a summary of the abnormalities is given in Table 3. Seven patients had normal CT scans. The five with reported abnormalities are summarized in Table 4. Anticonvulsants being taken when the decline was noted are described in Table

Table 2.   Seizure classification

Patient	Tonic-clinic	Absence	Complex Partial	Myoclonic
1	*	*		
2	*	*	*	*
3	*	*	*	
4	*	*		
5			*	
6	*			*
7	*			
8			*	
9	*	*	*	
10	*	*		*
11	*		*	
12	*	*		*

Table 3.   EEG abnormalities

Generalized non-specific abnormalities	2
Localized non-specific abnormalities	1
Generalized epileptic abnormalities	8
Focal epileptic abnormalities	1

Table 4.   CT abnormalities

Patient	Age	Sex	Abnormality
2	19	M	R temporal horn enlargement
3	22	M	R Sylvian Fissure wider than left
7	36	M	R temporal horn enlargement
8	34	M	Widening of sulci in both parietal lobes
10	19	F	Bilateral enlargement of anterior horns and bodies of lateral ventricles

Table 5.   Anticonvulsants being taken when deterioration noted

Patient	DPH	CBZ	NaV	Prim	Clon
1		*	*		
2	*	*	*		
3		*	*		
4	*	*		*	*
5			*		*
6		*	*		
7		*		*	
8		*			*
9	*				
10		*			
11		*	*		
12		*	*		

DPH = phenytoin, CBZ = carbamazepine, NaV = sodium valproate, Prim = primidone, Clon = clonazepam.

5, and all anticonvulsants ever taken are shown in Table 6. These probably represent general prescribing habits. Ten patients were on more than one drug at the time the intellectual decline was noted. There was no history of alcohol abuse or criminal record in any subject.

There was no significant abnormality recorded in serum electrolytes, liver function tests, calcium, vitamin B12, folate, red cell folate, full blood count or thyroid function tests, and there was no record of anticonvulsant toxicity. Syphilitic serology was negative in all cases.

Table 6. All anticonvulsants ever taken

Patient	PB	DPH	CBZ	NaV	Prim	Clon	Etho
1		*	*	*			
2	*	*	*	*	*		*
3	*	*	*	*		*	
4		*	*	*	*	*	
5		*					
6	*			*	*		
7	*		*	*	*		*
8	*		*	*	*	*	
9		*					
10		*	*	*			
11		*	*	*			
12	*		*	*	*	*	

PB = phenobarbitone, DPH = phenytoin, CBZ = carbamazepine, NaV = sodium valproate, Prim = primidone, Clon = clonazepam, Etho = ethosuximide.

Clinical assessment of current mental state revealed no abnormality other than intellectual impairment in five cases. Patient 3 showed obvious organic impairment of the mental state with disorientation, and patients 9 and 4 showed neurotic symptoms. Patient 8 displayed psychotic symptoms during post-ictal states, and patient 1 showed evidence of a schizoid personality.

In patients 11 and 12, both female, the intellectual decline had apparently been reversed following a change in medication, in one case following selective withdrawal of sodium valproate from a polytherapy regime, and in other case following cessation of all anticonvulsant medication (carbamazepine and sodium valproate).

From that small series it did seem as if intellectual deterioration could occur in epilepsy, although apparently very rarely, and if there were to be a true syndrome related to the epilepsy itself rather than its treatment it might be more likely to occur in males with a long history of poorly controlled epilepsy, showing more than one clinical seizure type, with diffuse generalized EEG abnormalities. From such a small sample it was not possible to further elucidate the nature of the cognitive deficit.

SECOND STUDY

At the David Lewis Centre, we have carried out more systematic studies. We have ensured that all admissions to our assessment unit are given as comprehensive a psychological test battery as possible, including the NART (Nelson, 1982) the WAIS, and a series of neuropsychological tests. We have found very substantial evidence for intellectual deterioration in a large number of subjects, and I shall now discuss some of our results in more detail.

Nelson (1982) used current reading ability (assessed on the National Adult Reading Test and Schonell) to predict 'premorbid' Wechsler Adult Intelligence Scale (WAIS) Full Scale IQ in patients with dementia. Nelson's procedures were adopted in the present study. Full Scale IQ (FSIQ) was estimated from reading scores using her tables and her recommeded short version of the WAIS was used to obtain current IQs. Predicted-Observed FSIQ discrepancies were compared with Nelson's normal standardization sample, and those large enough to be recorded by <5% of normals were taken as indicating the presence of intellectual deterioration (corresponding discrepancy sizes >13 points and >12 points for subjects with predicted FSIQ >86 and 74–85 respectively.)

It is reasonable to assume that individuals identified by this procedure will be 'true positives'. However, the parallel assumption, that subjects not meeting the criteria for deterioration have not declined is unreasonable. The procedure may lead to misclassification of subjects who experienced difficulties with reading acquisition (shown to be associated with epilepsy in children, e.g. Rutter et al., 1970) and of subjects whose present cognitive impairment disrupts reading skills. Therefore in our present study, the 'deteriorated' subjects are considered to be a valid subset of the intellectually deteriorated population. The 'Control' subjects (with smaller Predicted-Observed IQ discrepancies) probably represent a heterogeneous group, most of whom have not deteriorated, but some of whom have declined.

Nature and extent of the cognitive deficit

The FSIQ represents the standing of the individual with respect to his or her age peers in terms of his Full Scale Total Score. This latter is a composite of scores on up to eleven subtests which were designed to assess diverse cognitive abilities. Therefore a lowering of FSIQ could reflect some deterioration in all subtest scores or severe decline in only one or two. In this study, deterioration in Vocabulary (V) and Block Design (BD) scores was investigated as these subtests have the highest loadings on the two most influential group factors arising in factor analyses of the WAIS in normals. They are accepted as tapping verbal comprehension and perceptual organization abilities (Cohen, 1957).

Subjects

The subjects were all residents at the David Lewis Centre for Epilepsy. They were either undergoing an assessment admission or were longer-stay residents. All had severe epilepsy, with partial seizures plus or minus secondary generalization and had been treated with a variety of anti-epileptic drugs. Only those also fulfilling the following criteria were included: age <50 years; predicted FSIQ >74; Schonell Graded Word Reading Test Score >50 correct; no

Table 7. Age, predicted FSIQ, obtained FSIQ and Predicted-Obtained discrepancy

		Deteriorated males N = 10	Deteriorated females N = 10	'Control' females N = 10
Age (years)	mean	36.1	34.6	33.6
	range	24–42	20–43	19–45
Predicted FSIQ	mean	99.4	102.5	94.6
	range	84–106	90–119	81–114
Obtained FSIQ	mean	75.1	82.8	91.3
	range	63–91	65–104	80–108
Predicted-Obtained	mean	24.3	19.70	3.3
Discrepancy	range	16–33	15–25	–5–7

evidence of severe head injury in adult life; no record of alcohol abuse in the notes. Suitable subjects were identified either through routine neuropsychological assessment of all new admissions or through assessment as part of an ongoing survey of existing adult residents. The first ten males and ten females identified as showing intellectual deterioration (as defined above) were included in the study. Subsequently a 'control' group of ten women with smaller Predicted–Observed discrepancies was selected so that it was balanced for age with the deteriorated female group. The mean age, predicted and obtained IQs are given in Table 7.

Method

A short version of the WAIS comprising Arithmetic, Similarities, Digit Span, Vocabulary, Picture Completion, Block Design and Picture Arrangement subtests was used to estimate current FSIQ. Vocabulary (V) and Block Design (BD) subtest scores were converted to age-scaled scores and these were used as estimates of current ability. Previous level of score on these subtests was assumed to be reflected in the Predicted FSIQ. Significant discrepancies between Predicted FSIQ and age-scaled scores were taken to indicate deterioration in the latter scores.

Results

Predicted FSIQs and V and BD age-scaled scores were converted to T scores (which have a normal distribution, mean 50; SD 10) to make direct comparison possible. A subtest T score of >10 points lower than an IQ T score was defined as denoting deterioration in that subtest score. Table 8 gives the frequency of deteriorated subtest scores for the ten male and ten female deteriorated subjects. It can be seen from this that five subjects showed deterioration in both

Table 8.   Frequency of deteriorated subtest scores for the two deteriorated groups

	Deteriorated males	Deteriorated females	Total
Subtest deteriorated			
Neither	0	1	1
V only	1	5	6
BD only	5	3	8
Both	4	1	5
	10	10	20

subtest scores, 6 in V only, 8 in BD and 1 in neither. It is also apparent that the sexes were comparable in showing decline in V score (5 male, 6 female) but differed significantly (p <0.05 Fisher's Exact Test) in decline in BD score (9 males, 4 female). Only one of the ten 'control' females showed subtest deterioration. She declined on BD alone.

Discussion

This study involved small numbers of subjects so that the following conclusions are best considered as being in need of replication and further research.

The finding that an albeit far from optimal group of female 'control' subjects who showed only one instance of subtest deterioration provides some justification for the assumption that V and BD decline is a characteristic of subjects showing intellectual deterioration rather than of all people with epilepsy. The results obtained from the 20 deteriorated subjects indicated that although deterioration was generalized (i.e. apparent in two specific subtests) for some subjects, the majority showed subtest specific decline. Therefore intellectual deterioration in people with epilepsy does not appear to arise from a generalized reduction of all cognitive abilities but rather from a selective impairment of some.

The presence of a sex difference in terms of the subtests showing deterioration suggests that males and females may be affected differently and that the sexes should be treated separately in future research.

LOCUS OF IMPAIRMENT OF COGNITIVE FUNCTIONING (PRELIMINARY STUDY OF FEMALES)

The presence of specific impairment of cognitive ability suggests that there may be corresponding selective impairment of cortical functioning. I shall now describe a preliminary attempt to identify those cortical areas which show impaired functioning by comprehensive neuropsychological assessment.

Subjects

Eight of the ten women in the deteriorated group of the previous study were available for neuropsychological assessment (two had left the Centre; age 38 and 43, duration of epilepsy 34 and 36 years). Eight of the original control females were chosen from the original ten to be balanced with the deteriorated subjects with respect to age. Twelve of the sixteen subjects were right-handed, one showed mixed handedness, two were left-handed and in one, left-handedness was forced by a right hemiplegia which had been present from birth.

Method

A battery of seven neuropsychological tests was used. The tests and the cortical areas that they are believed to tap are given in Table 9. The tests do not allow good discrimination between left and right frontal lobe functioning and in a few cases between left and right anterior temporal lobe functioning. For each test, a cut-off score for 'impairment' was derived from available normative data. This allowed a profile of impairment to be constructed for each subject.

Table 9.   Neuropsychological test battery and cortical areas tapped

Cortical area	Tests
Frontal lobes	Modified Wisconsin Card sorting (MW) Verbal fluency (VF)
Left anterior temporal	Wechsler Logical Memory delayed recall (LM) Token test (TT)
Left posterior temporal and/or parietal	Facial recognition (FR)
Right anterior temporal	Rey-Osterrieth (RO)
Right posterior temporal and/or parietal	Judgement of line orientation (JLO)

Results

One deteriorated subject was not tested on the Rey-Osterrieth and one on the Modified Wisconsin. Each subject's score on each test was classified as impaired or not impaired according to the cut-offs that had been defined. Impairment of functioning of a cortical area was recorded as present if the score on at least one test designed to tap it was impaired. Left hemisphere dominance was assumed for all subjects. Table 10 shows the resulting impairment profiles for the eight deteriorated subjects and the eight 'controls'.

The 'control' subjects appear to be heterogeneous as was expected from the use of current reading ability to predict IQ. One obtained no impaired scores.

Table 10　Neuropsychological test impairment profiles

Cortical area	Test	Deteriorated								'Control'							
		1	2	3	4	5	6	7	8	9	10	11	12	13	14	15	16
Frontal	VF			·		·	·	·									·
	MW	·			—											·	
L Ant Temp	TT	·		·	·	·										·	·
	LM			·	·	·										·	·
L Post Temp/Par	FR	·	·		·		·									o	o
R Ant Temp	RO	·	—	·	θ	·	θ					·	·	·			
R Post Temp/Par	JLO					·		·				·		·			·

· = impaired test score.
θ = low RO score may reflect extensive left temporal lobe *not* right temporal lobe impairment.
o = Left posterior temporal/parietal lobe impairment may be being masked by right posterior temporal/parietal impairment.
— = NA.

Two of them (subjects 15 and 16) showed patterns of impairment which are very similar to those obtained by the majority of the deteriorated subjects. The impairment profiles of the other five (nos 9–13) whilst similar to each other were quite different from those of the deteriorated subjects.

Although there is some obvious circularity of argument, it is tempting to conclude that subjects 9–14 represent the true non-deteriorated subjects, whilst subjects 15 and 16 are misclassified deteriorated subjects. If this is assumed to be the case, it becomes clear that deteriorated subjects are distinguished from controls by the presence of impairment of functioning of frontal and/or left temporal (and possibly left parietal) lobes. It is possible that intellectual deterioration, defined in terms of decline in IQ, is attributable to impairment of functioning of some or all of these cortical areas. Of course, this is speculative and requires appropriate investigation with larger numbers of subjects, more adequate control subjects, and non-cognitive evaluation of cortical functioning.

DISCUSSION AND CONCLUSIONS

One feature of our studies at the David Lewis Centre had been a difficulty in finding male control subjects, which is why the neuropsychological test battery results have so far only been discussed for females. It did seem that in our highly selected population of people with severe epilepsy referred to a special centre (where the referral sex ratio is approximately 50 : 50 with perhaps a slight preponderance to males) that the males are at much higher risk of having had significant cognitive deterioration than females. Whether the pattern of that deterioration involves a selective dominant hemisphere fronto-temporal impairment in males is not clear, but the WAIS subtest analysis referred to earlier certainly raises the possibility that there might be a sex difference. Our male subjects were generally so impaired as to be outside the standardization range of the neuropsychological tests, so we have not yet been able to address this problem with a large enough sample, although the work continues and we hope to be able to report some results in the near future.

The consequences of fronto-temporal dysfunction are however worth pondering for a moment. These extend beyond the realm of cognitive functioning alone.

Damage to the orbitofrontal region of the frontal lobe is associated with disinhibited impulsive behaviour, the so-called 'pseudopsychopathic syndrome', in which cognitive impairment may not be a feature, while a more extensive lesion involving the dorsolateral frontal lobe may produce profound slowing of thought and action with difficulty in initiating intentional action, distinguished from retarded depressive illness only by the lack of the characteristic mood change, the 'pseudodepressed syndrome'. The two syndromes may coexist.

There has been a great deal of speculation about the effects of temporal lobe dysfunction on personality and behaviour, in particular in the interictal personality characteristics found in temporal lobe epilepsy. Some authors refer to a syndrome of personality change caused by excessive discharges in the limbic system (Bear and Fedio, 1977; Brown, 1982; Roberts, 1984) which contains most of the elements of the 'epileptic personality' described by nineteenth- and early twentieth-century authors, such as emotional lability, hyposexuality and a tendency to adhere to each thought feeling and action, so-called 'thought viscosity'. This latter would obviously affect cognitive processes. Unfortunately, it is not easy to tease out the relative contributions of seizures, subclinical seizure discharges or associated brain damage from the psychosocial effects of a seizure disorder, and of course, all these factors interact with chronic anticonvulsant effects.

In our female group, a dorsolateral frontal lobe syndrome in association with dominant hemisphere temporal lobe dysfunction could well produce a clinical picture akin to a dementia syndrome. The question arises why this pattern should appear at all. To attempt an answer would be beyond the scope of this chapter except that I would like to end by drawing attention to the relationship between discrete neuropsychological impairment and neurophysiological abnormalities. In a different study (Brown & Vaughan, 1986) we compared the neuropsychological test impairment profiles of a number of patients with epilepsy with the results of EEG and Topographical Brain Mapping and found a significant correlation. Psychological impairment was topographically related to neurophysiological phenomena such as spike foci and areas of excessive slow wave activity. What we might be seeing is a pattern of cognitive impairment contributed to by abnormal interictal EEG activity which provides a clinical picture resembling dementia.

REFERENCES

BEAR, D. and FEDIO, P. (1977) Quantitative analysis of interictal behaviour in temporal lobe epilepsy. *Arch. Neurol.*, **34**, 454–467.

BERKLEY, H.J. (1901) *A Treatise on Mental Diseases*. Henry Kimpton, London.

BROWN, S.W. (1982) Epilepsy and Psychotherapy. In LOPES, G. (ed.) *Progressos Em Terapeutica Psiquiátrica*, pp. 131–160. Biblioteca do Hospital do Conde de Ferreira.

BROWN, S.W. and ABEYASINGHE, R. (1984) Is there an epileptic dementia? *Acta Neurol. Scand.*, **70**, 233.

BROWN, S.W. and REYNOLDS, E.H. (1981) Cognitive impairment in epileptic patients. In *Epilepsy and Psychiatry* (eds E.H. REYNOLDS and M.R. TRIMBLE) Churchill-Livingstone, London.

BROWN, S.W. and VAUGHAN, M. (1986) Topographical Brain Mapping and neuropsychological dysfunction in adult patients with epilepsy. Poster presented at British-Danish-Dutch Epilepsy Symposium, York.

COHEN, J. (1957) The factorial structure of the WAIS between early adulthood and old age. *J. Consult. Psychol.*, **21**, 283–390.

DAWSON, S. and CONN, J.C.M. (1929) The intelligence of epileptic children. *Arch. Dis. Child.*, **4**, 142–151.

DELANEY, R.C., ROSEN, A.J., MATTSON, R.H. and NOVELLY, R.A. (1980) Memory function in focal epilepsy: a comparison of non-surgical unilateral temporal lobe and frontal lobe samples. *Cortex,* **16**, 103–117.

FETTERMAN, J. and BARNES, R.R. (1934) Serial studies of the intelligence of patients with epilepsy. *Neuropsychologica,* **7**, 287–300.

GOWERS, W.R. (1881) *Epilepsy and other Chronic Convulsive Disease*. Churchill, London.

KUGELMASS, I.N., POULL, L.E. and RUDNICK, J. (1938) Mental growth of epileptic children. *Am. J. Dis. Child.*, **55**, 295–303.

MAUDSLEY, H. (1874) *Responsibility in Mental Disease*. Appleton, New York.

NELSON, H.E. (1982) *National Adult Reading Test. Test Manual*. NFER-Nelson.

PATTERSON, H.A. and FONNER, D. (1928) Some observations on the intelligence quotient in epileptics. *Psychiat. Quart.*, **31**, 542–548.

ROBERTS, J.K.A. (1984) *Differential Diagnosis in Neuropsychiatry*. John Wiley, Chichester.

RUTTER, M., GRAHAM, P. and YULE, W. (1970) *A Neuropsychiatric Study in Childhood*. Spastics International Medical Publications.

SULLIVAN, E.B. and GAHAGAN, L. (1935) On intelligence of epileptic children. *Genet. Psychol. Monogr.*, **17**, 309–375.

14

Late onset seizures and dementia: a review of epidemiology and aetiology

SIMON D. SHORVON
National Hospitals for Nervous Diseases and Institute of Neurology, London

INTRODUCTION

Both dementia and epilepsy are common in late life, and yet surprisingly, there has been little direct research concerned either with epilepsy in dementing illnesses, or the problems of dementia in patients with epilepsy. In this chapter, the epidemiology and the main causes of epilepsy and dementia in the elderly will be outlined, and the commonest causes of the association of the two conditions discussed. It is important to establish the cause of epilepsy in the elderly, and all such patients require adequate investigation. The extent of investigation of dementia depends on clinical circumstances, and dementia is treatable in only a minority of patients (about 7% of cases referred to hospital; Marsden, 1985). In contrast, late onset seizures are usually successfully treated in the majority of patients. Dementia may also develop in a small proportion of patients with epilepsy. This is usually after a long history of epilepsy, in young patients and in patients with severe epilepsy. The cause of the dementia is often unclear and several factors may be responsible. This 'epileptic dementia' will not be presented further here, but has been discussed in Chapter 13.

EPIDEMIOLOGY

Dementia in the elderly

Studies of the prevalence of dementia suggest that about 10% of the population over the age of 65 years exhibit some degree of dementia, and that in about 50% of these cases, the dementia is severe (Kay et al., 1970; Wells, 1979). The prevalence increases with age, and is over 20% in those over 80 years of age. Thus in the UK, over 750,000 elderly persons are affected by dementia. The prognosis of dementia is poor; the mean life expectancy is about 2.5 years, compared with about 9–11 years in a matched population without dementia. Surveys have also suggested prevalence rates of between 2–15% of borderline dementia, and in a small follow-up study (over three years), about 30% of such cases developed full-blown dementia, about 30% were unchanged and 30% were regarded as normal when seen again (Kay et al., 1970). There are no figures giving the proportion of demented patients in a population who also have epilepsy.

Epilepsy in the elderly

It has been previously held that epilepsy is uncommon in old age. It is certainly true that the epilepsy developing in childhood and adult life has usually remitted by late adult life. In studies from Rochester, Minnesota (Annegers et al., 1979) and Tonbridge, Kent (Goodridge and Shorvon, 1983), it has been shown that about 50% of all cases of epilepsy develop before the age of 20, and that 60–70% of cases have entered long-term remission within fifteen years or so of the onset of epilepsy. The incidence of epilepsy falls in middle life, but rises steeply again in late life, and preliminary findings from the *National General Practice Study of Epilepsy* (a cohort study of newly diagnosed cases), for instance, show that about 20% of new cases of epilepsy start after the age of 50 (unpublished data). As populations in developed countries age, the problems of epilepsy in late life will become more prominent. At a best approximation, the annual incidence rate of epilepsy in patients older than 50 years is about 60/100,000 persons, and in the UK therefore there will be about 4500 new cases of epilepsy a year in this age group. The prevalence of epilepsy in the elderly in the UK is about 5–10/1000, and there will therefore be about 35–75,000 elderly persons with epilepsy in the country. A number of these epileptic patients will also have dementia, but the exact proportion is not known.

Aetiology of dementia and epilepsy in elderly patients

Some causes of dementia and late onset epilepsy are listed in Table 1. A precise aetiological classification for dementia may be difficult in life, and many degenerative diseases can be identified with certainty only by pathological examination. Nevertheless, the clinical presentations of the commonest dementing illnesses are sufficiently distinct for a reasonably secure provisional diagnosis to be made in most cases. Using clinical and pathological criteria, Alzheimer's disease probably accounts for between 50–60% of all cases of dementia, vascular disease for about 20–30% and other causes for a further

Table 1. Causes of dementia and epilepsy in adults

Primary cerebral degenerative disorders
  Alzheimer's disease
  Huntington's disease
  Wilson's disease

Degenerative cerebrovascular disorders
  Multi-infarct dementia
  Cerebral infarction
  Lacunar infarction
  Cerebral arteritis
  Binswanger's disease

Other cerebrovascular disorders
  Subdural haematoma
  Other intracranial haemmorhage
  Giant aneurysms
  Cardiac disorders
  Angioma

Cerebral infections and inflammation
  Creutzfeldt–Jacob disease
  Bacterial meningitis
  Tuberculous meningitis
  Neurosyphilis
  Whipple's disease
  Viral encephalitis
  Cerebral abscess
  Behçet's disease
  Multiple sclerosis

Trauma (open and closed head injury)

Intracranial tumours (benign and malignant)

Alcoholism

Miscellaneous
  Metabolic (e.g. uraemia, hepatic disease, hypocapnia, porphyria, hypocalcaemia,
    hypoglycaemia)
  Deficiency disease (e.g. pellagra, B12 deficiency)
  Drugs and poisons
  Inherited diseases (e.g. Leigh's disease, Kuf's disease, metachromatic
    leucodystrophy)

10–20%. Cerebrovascular disease is also increasingly recognized as the major causal factor of epilepsy in the elderly, accounting perhaps for about 30–50% of all cases. Cerebral tumour accounts for about 10–15% of cases of late onset epilepsy, other mass lesions (e.g. subdural haematoma) for about 5%, alcohol or drug-induced seizures for a further 5–10%, and other causes are rare. In about 30% of cases no cause is identified, although in many of these patients the seizures will be due to occult cerebrovascular disease.

In demented patients with epilepsy, therefore, the most common underlying cause is degenerative cerebrovascular disease, although other conditions such as the primary dementing illnesses, alcohol, tumour, trauma, and cerebral infection may account for a small number of cases. The other causes listed in Table 1 are rare.

Degenerative cerebrovascular disease

Multi-infarct dementia is the commonest vascular cause of dementia. The degree of dementia depends both on the size and position of infarction. Thus, usually only large cortical infarcts cause dementia, but small strategically placed deep infarcts may have profound cognitive effects. Although 'arterio-sclerosis' has in the past been thought to be an important cause of dementia, it is now clear that arteriosclerosis per se seldom causes significant intellectual impairment, and dementia implies more extensive vascular disease. Dementia may also be associated with the leuco-encephalopathy of hypertensive vascular disease (Binswanger's disease), and with the less common vascular pathology (e.g. congophilic angiopathy, cerebral arteritis).

For over a hundred years, it has been recognized that degenerative cerebro-vascular disease may cause epilepsy. In 1864, Hughlings Jackson observed that 'it is not very uncommon to find when a patient has recovered or is recovering from hemiplegia, the result of embolism of the middle cerebral artery or of some branch of this vessel, that he is attacked by convulsions beginning in some part of the paralysed region' (see Jackson, 1931). In 1881, Gowers reported 66 cases of hemiplegia and epilepsy and introduced the term 'post-hemiplegic epilepsy'. In recent years, cerebrovascular disease has been established as the most common identifiable cause of late onset epilepsy.

Epilepsy may be the initial or only clinical manifestation of cerebrovascular disease. In a case control study of CT from the National Hospitals, Queen Square in 132 patients presenting with epilepsy developing after the age of 40 as the only neurological feature, unexpected vascular lesions were found in 15 patients and two controls (p=0.003, Fisher's exact test). In this series, lacunar infarction was found in ten cases, cerebral infarction in six (one patient having both lacunar and cerebral infarction) (Roberts et al., 1987). Shinton et al. (1987) analysed the previous history of 230 patients presenting with stroke to a general hospital, and found a significantly higher instance of epilepsy preceding the stroke than in case controls (although a similar report by Frisher and Herishanu (1987) found no excess of epilepsy). In the National Hospitals study, ischaemic lesions were commoner in older patients, and in those with systemic vascular disease. In further studies in these patients, the incidence of vascular lesions shown on MRI is significantly greater than those shown on CT, and MRI will prove a more sensitive method of diagnosis of vascular disease than CT. On the evidence of these studies, it seems likely that in at least 20% (and possibly more) of patients presenting with 'idiopathic' late onset epilepsy, the epilepsy will be due to occult vascular disease.

Epilepsy is also common after acute stroke. In a post mortem study from the Massachusetts General Hospital of 104 brains with evidence of cerebral infarction, a history of seizures was obtained retrospectively in 12.5% (compared with 2.7% of patients with cerebral arteriosclerosis without infarction) (Richardson and Dodge, 1954). In this investigation, it was noted that cortical infarction was more commonly associated with epilepsy than subcortical infarction, and this observation has been confirmed in subsequent studies. Perhaps 15% of patients presenting with a first seizure after the age of 25 will have a history of previous stroke (Dam et al., 1985; Lopez et al., 1985), and a third of patients presenting with the onset of epilepsy after the age of 60.

Epilepsy may also occur in the acute phase of stroke only, and indeed may be the presenting symptom of stroke, but only a proportion of these cases progress to chronic epilepsy. In a review of seven studies of epilepsy and vascular disease, Lesser et al. (1985) found that in the 231 reported cases, about two-thirds had focal seizures and one-third generalized seizures.

The proportion of cases of vascular epilepsy with dementia is unclear. Probably about 20% of patients with vascular dementia will have epilepsy, and syncope is also common (Lishman, 1978).

Epilepsy in the primary cerebral degenerative disorders

Alzheimer's disease is the commonest dementing illness encountered in elderly populations, yet surprisingly there are no large series reporting the prevalence or characteristics of epilepsy in this population. Data from small or selected reports suggest that epilepsy occurs in about 25–33%. The epilepsy is usually mild and the seizures infrequent, and epilepsy is a problem particularly in the terminal stages of the disease (Radermecker, 1974). The incidence of EEG changes is much higher, but these do not usually have specific epileptic features.The EEG may be low amplitude, with a reduction of alpha rhythm, and with diffuse theta and delta components. These EEG changes are usually much more marked than in other primary dementias. Pick's disease rarely causes seizures.

In Huntington's disease epilepsy is also uncommon, probably occurring in about 5%, again without any specific features. It has been said to be commoner in juvenile onset Huntington's disease and in the rigid forms than in the classic syndrome. The EEG is frequently abnormal showing changes similar to those in Alzheimer's disease, although these are usually less marked.

In Creutzfeldt–Jakob disease, epilepsy is common both in the early stages and in the established disease. Myoclonus occurs in over 80% of cases, either as rapid repeated contractions of a muscle or muscle group in the face or limbs, or more massive contractions of a whole limb (Will and Matthews, 1984). The myoclonus may be startle responsive. Other generalized or simple or complex partial seizures occur in about 10% of cases, and are usually infrequent. Seizures are rare in the terminal stages of the condition, and even the myoclonus, which may be profound in the established condition, tends to diminish or disappear in the terminal stages. The EEG in established Creutzfeldt–Jakob disease is often very abnormal, and is of great diagnostic value, but the changes are often not present in the early stages. The alpha rhythm may disappear, and the record can be dominated by repetitive and generalized spike or spike-wave discharges, which may show biphasic or triphasic patterns.

In Wilson's disease, epilepsy occurs in about 5% of cases. Seizures may occur at any stage of the disease, and indeed may be the presenting symptom. Often the epilepsy begins soon after treatment is started. The seizures may be partial or generalized and are often frequent and severe, but the response to treatment is usually good. The mechanism of the seizures has been recently studied, and some cases may be due to penicillamine induced pyridoxine deficiency, although a direct effect of copper deposition is probably responsible for most cases.

Alcohol, epilepsy and dementia

The relationship of seizures and dementia to alcoholism is complex, and there are several distinct causal factors which complicate any investigation or evaluation (Brennan and Lyttle, 1987). Seizures are classically associated with alcohol withdrawal. For instance, of the seizures in 241 patients described by Victor and Brausch (1967), 213 occurred on withdrawal. In 100 of these 241 patients, there was only a single seizure, and about 50% of the withdrawal seizures occurred within 13–24 hours after cessation of drinking. The seizures are usually generalized and the EEG may show photosensitivity.

Epilepsy unrelated to withdrawal may also occur in alcoholics, either due to the direct toxic effects of alcohol or to associated head injury, drug intake or other established cerebral disorders. In a large series of 1421 alcoholic patients admitted to hospitals in the Feltre area in 1981, the incidence of epilepsy was about 10% (Devetag et al., 1983). About one third of these cases were classified as 'alcoholic epilepsy', in which the seizures were recurrent, not related to withdrawal or bout drinking, and not due to any other identifiable cause. About 20% of the cases of epilepsy in this population had other potential causes identified (usually trauma or vascular disease). In 25% of patients in a recent series of late onset epilepsies attending a general hospital, alcohol withdrawal was the main cause (Dam et al., 1985), and alcohol misuse was the sole precipitating factor in 20% of the cases of status epilepticus reported by Pilke et al. (1984).

Alcoholism may also complicate established epilepsy, and in a series of admissions with epilepsy to a state hospital in Denver, 41% of patients abused alcohol and the seizures were precipitated by alcohol in 24% (Earnest and Yurnell, 1976).

Dementia in alcoholism can result from a variety of causes. It may be the result of Wernicke-Korsakoff syndrome (due to thiamine deficiency), in which the major pathological damage is found bilaterally in the mamillary bodies, the medial thalamic nuclei, the periaqueductal region and the tegmentum of the pons and the medulla. In lesions confined to these areas, epilepsy is unlikely to be common. Coexistent cortical damage is frequent, however, and is often epileptogenic. Alcoholic dementia may also result from pellagratous cerebral damage, Marchiafava-Bignami disease, and acquired hepatocerebral degeneration, and in these conditions epilepsy may occur although is seldom a leading clinical feature. Alcoholism may also result in secondary cerebral disease, due for instance to trauma, cerebrovascular disease, acute or chronic hepatic disease; and all these conditions may be complicated by the occurrence of severe epilepsy.

The frequency and clinical features of 'primary alcoholic dementia', distinct from Wernicke-Korsakoff syndrome has been the subject of some controversy. Most cases of so-called alcoholic dementia are due to the Wernicke-Korsakoff syndrome, and the concept of primary dementia due to alcoholism is rather ill-defined (see Victor and Adams, 1985). There are no studies of the incidence of epilepsy in patients with alcoholic dementia.

Other conditions causing dementia and epilepsy in the elderly

Cerebral tumours account for about 10–20% of all cases of late onset epilepsy. In one series of 139 cases of cerebral tumour manifested by epilepsy of late onset, 45% were malignant gliomas, 25% metastases, and 17% meningiomas (Sheehan, 1958). Although this was a selected series of patients, referred to a neurosurgical unit, it is worth stressing that about one fifth of the tumours were benign. The site and size of the tumours are more important than the histology in determining the propensity to cause seizures, and those in the temporal or frontal cortex are appreciably more epileptogenic than others.

In a personal series of 337 patients with histologically proven cerebral gliomas, referred to the National Hospitals, 59% had epilepsy. This was usually the first sign of cerebral disturbance and in all but three cases seizures had occurred by the time of initial presentation (see Shorvon, 1985).

About 5% of all cases presenting primarily as a dementing illness in adult life are found to have a cerebral tumour, although over 50% of patients with tumours will also manifest mental changes as the condition evolves. As is the case with epilepsy, it is the site, size and speed of development of the tumour which affect its propensity to cause dementia rather than the histological type.

Cerebral trauma is a potent cause of epilepsy, although it accounts for only a small proportion of cases of epilepsy in the elderly (less than 5%). Early epilepsy occurs in about 5% of patients admitted to hospital with head injury, and about one quarter of these cases will continue to have seizures. Epilepsy is more likely to occur in open rather than closed head injuries, in injuries complicated by intracranial haematomas or depressed skull fracture and in those cases with a prolonged period of post-traumatic amnesia (Jennett, 1987). Epilepsy after head injury is most likely to develop within 12 months of the injury, although there is a small risk of epilepsy over subsequent years. Post-traumatic seizures have focal features in about 50% of cases. The elderly are at particular risk from subdural haematomas, and cerebral damage is also more likely to occur after falling. Dementia may also result from major head trauma. For head-injured patients classified as 'severe' (Glasgow Coma Scale <8), about 50% will die. Of the survivors, 5% will remain in a persistent vegetative state, 20% have severe disability, and only 35% will recover with an IQ in the normal range and without specific cognitive defects (Jennett et al., 1977). The elderly head-injured patient fares worse than the young. Mild head injury also may result in more subtle forms of dementia. Intracranial haemorrhages (especially subdural haemorrhages) are also a potent cause of dementia in the elderly.

Cerebral infection may result in severe epilepsy and dementia. Brain abscess may result in epilepsy in about three-quarters of survivors, and dementia in a significant proportion of these cases. Bacterial meningitis causes epilepsy in about 5% of cases, and cognitive impairment in about 10%. Tuberculous meningitis frequently causes seizures and cognitive deficits and mild to moderate neurological impairment is seen in between 30–60% of cases. Severe encephalitis (usually due to herpes simplex (type 1) virus in the UK) causes severe epilepsy in the majority of survivors and significant cognitive deficit in over 50%.

REFERENCES

ANNEGERS, J.F., HAUSER, W.A. and ELVEBACK, L.R. (1979) Remission of seizures and relapse in patients with epilepsy. *Epilepsia*, **20**, 729–737.

BRENNAN, F.N. and LYTTLE, J.A. (1987) Alcohol and seizures: a review. *J. Roy. Soc. Med.*, **80**, 571–573.

DAM, A.M., FUGLSANG-FREDERIKSEN, A., SVARRE-OLSEN, U. and DAM, M. (1985) Late onset epilepsy: etiologies, types of seizure, and value of clinical investigation, EEG and computerized tomography scan. *Epilepsia*, **26**, 227–231.

DEVETAG, F., MANDICH, G., ZAIOTTI, G., TOFFOLO, G.G. (1983) Alcoholic epilepsy:

review of cases and proposed classification and etiopathogenesis. *Ital. J. Med. Sci.*, **3**, 275–284.

EARNEST, M.P. and YARNELL, P.R. (1976) Seizure admissions to a city hospital: the role of alcohol. *Epilepsia*, **17**, 387–393.

FRISHER, S. and HERISHANU, Y.U. (1987) Frequency of epilepsy preceding stroke. *Lancet*, **ii**, 393.

GOODRIDGE, D.G.M. and SHORVON, S.D. (1983) Epileptic seizures in a population of 6000: treatment and prognosis. *Br. Med. J.*,**287**, 645–747.

GOWERS, W.R. (1881) *Epilepsy and Other Chronic Convulsive Disorders: Their Causes, Symptoms and Treatment.* Churchill, London.

JACKSON, J.H. (1931) On the scientific and empirical investigation of the epilepsies. In J. TAYLOR (ed.) *Selected Writings of John Hughlings Jackson.* Hodder and Stoughton, London.

JENNETT, B. (1987) Epilepsy after head injury and intracranial surgery. In A. HOPKINS (ed.) *Epilepsy*, pp. 401–411. Chapman and Hall, London.

JENNETT, B., TEASDALE, G., GALBRAITH, S., PICHARD, J., GRANT, H., BRAAKMAN, R., AVEZAAT, C., MAAS, A., MINDERHOUD, J., VECHT, C.J., HEIDEN, J., SMALL, R., CATON, W. and KURTZE, T. (1977) Severe head injuries in three countries. *J. Neurol. Neurosurg. Psychiatry*, **40**, 291–298.

KAY, D.W.K., BEAMISH, P. and ROTH, M. (1964) Old age mental disorders in Newcastle upon Tyne, part 1: a study of prevalence. *Br. J. Psych.*, **110**, 146–158.

KAY, D.W., BERGMANN, K., FOSTER, E.M., McKECHNIE, A.A. and ROTH, M. (1970) Mental illness and hospital usage in the elderly: a random sample follow up. *Comprehen. Psychiatry*, **11**, 26–35.

LESSER, R.P., LUDERS, H., DINNER, D.S. and MORRIS, H.H. (1985) Epileptic seizures due to thrombotic and embolic cerebrovascular disease in older patients. *Epilepsia*, **26**, 622–630.

LISHMAN, W.A. (1978) *Organic Psychiatry.* Blackwell Science Publications, Oxford.

LOPEZ, J.L.P., LONGO, J., QUINTANA, F., DIEZ, C. and BERCIANO, J. (1985) Late onset epileptic seizures. *Acta Neurol. Scand.*, **72**, 380–384.

MARSDEN, C.D. (1985) Dementia – assessment. In *Handbook of Clinical Neurology* 2 (**46**) *Neurobehavioural Disorders* (ed. J.A.M. FREDERIKS), pp. 221–232, Elsevier Science Publishers, Amsterdam.

PILKE, A., PARTINEN, M. and KOVANEN, J. (1984) Status epilepticus and alcohol abuse: an analysis of 82 status epilepticus admissions. *Acta Neurol. Scand.*, **70**, 443–450.

RADERMECKER, J. (1974) Epilepsy in the degenerative diseases. In *Handbook of Clinical Neurology* **15**: *The Epilepsies* (eds O. MAGNUS and A.M. LORENTZ DE HAAS), pp. 325–372, North-Holland, Amsterdam.

RICHARDSON, E.P. and DODGE, P.R. (1954) Epilepsy in cerebral vascular disease. *Epilepsia*, **3**, 49–65.

ROBERTS, R.C., SHORVON, S.D., COX, T.C.S. and GILLIATT, R.W. (1987) Silent infarction revealed by CT scanning in late onset epilepsy. *Epilepsia* (in press).

SHEEHAN, S. (1958) One thousand cases of late onset epilepsy. *Irish Med. J.*, 261–272.

SHINTON, R.A., GILL, J.S., ZEZULKA, A.S.V. and BEEVERS, D.G. (1987) The frequency of epilepsy preceding stroke: case control study in 230 patients. *Lancet*, **ii**, 11–12.

SHORVON, S.D. (1985) Late onset epilepsy. *Geriatric Med. Today*, **4**, 43–61.

VICTOR, M. and ADAMS, R.D. (1985) The alcoholic dementias. In *Handbook of Clinical Neurology* 2 (**46**): *Neurobehavioural Disorders* (ed. J.A.M. FREDERIKS), pp. 335–352. Elsevier Science Publishers, Amsterdam.

VICTOR, M. and BRAUSCH, C. (1967) The role of abstinence in the genesis of alcohol epilepsy. *Epilepsia*, **8**, 1–20.

WELLS, N.E.J. (1979) *Dementia in Old Age*. Office of Health Economics, London.
WILL, R.G. and MATTHEWS, W.B. (1984) A retrospective study of Creutzfeldt-Jacob disease in England and Wales 1970–1979: 1: Clinical features. *J. Neurol. Neurosurg. Psych.*, **47**, 134–140.

Discussion

Section V

Dr J. Duncan (Oxford): Dr Shorvon, in the patients who had alcohol-related epilepsy, had all of them had prior withdrawal seizures and could that be implicated?

Dr S.D. Shorvon: I do not know the answer. In the literature on alcohol and epilepsy there is a quite striking move away from the earlier preoccupation with withdrawal seizures. Now it is more a question of whether alcohol itself can cause brain damage.

Dr D.B. Smith: Dr Shorvon, you emphasized various aetiologies for seizures associated with alcoholism. Does that influence your therapeutic approach, recognizing that compliance may be a problem?

Dr S.D. Shorvon: I think that the treatment of epilepsy in a severe alcoholic is difficult, and in some cases no anticonvulsant treatment should be given. Alcohol withdrawal seizures need not require long-term anticonvulsant treatment although they may require short-term treatment.

Dr S.H. Green (Birmingham): Dr Loiseau, I am interested in how long does it take a child to show memory defects in the course of the disease?

Professor P. Loiseau: They can occur quite early. When a cognitive impairment is related to drug intake, it is two to three months before it begins to appear.

Dr S.H. Green: Is there any evidence that the younger the onset of epilepsy, the greater the deficit?

Professor P. Loiseau: Yes, it is clear.

Dr S.D. Shorvon: Professor Loiseau, how soon after the head injury were your patients assessed?

Professor P. Loiseau: The cognitive state of these severe head injury patients progresses rather rapidly, and then there is a plateau and they leave the rehabilitation centre at the beginning of the plateau. They were therefore tested when they were relatively stabilized.

199

Professor J. A. Corbett: Could I ask Dr Shorvon about the relationship between epilepsy and Alzheimer's disease? Some authors suggest seizures are very frequent in that condition.

Dr S. D. Shorvon: I am surprised that the incidence of epilepsy is said to be so high.

Professor R. C. Tallis (Salford): Can I pursue the question of the investigation of the patient with late onset epilepsy? There is a good case for doing a CT scan in the elderly who present with epilepsy and who are a reasonable prospect for surgery if a remedial lesion turns up. However, this view is not shared by everyone.

Dr S. D. Shorvon: We regularly pick up benign tumours in patients with late onset epilepsy who have no other suggestive features, either EEG or clinical.

Professor R. C. Tallis: But some people would say it was meddlesome to remove a meningioma in someone who presented with a fit and had no other neurological deficit.

Dr S. D. Shorvon: It depends a lot on the clinical situation, on the age, the size of the meningioma, and the general state of the patient.

Dr D. W. Chadwick: I have a lot of elderly patients with fits and meningiomas, and their meningiomas just do not change over the years. I am very resistant to letting surgeons loose on them.

Dr M. R. Trimble: Dr Brown, is there a specific pattern to the dementia you were discussing, as there is a specific pattern which allows us clinically to identify Alzheimer's disease or multi-infarct dementia with relative certainty?

Dr S. W. Brown: I feel that we will come up with something specific, but it is too early to say.

Dr M. R. Trimble: In a study which Dr Thompson and a number of other colleagues from the Chalfont Centre, including myself, carried out, we looked at a group of people who had undergone intellectual deterioration and a group who had not. Both had very extensive investigations, including CT scans, lumbar punctures, EEGs and psychometric testing. We also had a very thorough anamnesis of the total drug load that the patients had received for the past ten years, the total number of their seizures, and the total number of head injuries they had that needed stitching or medical attention. Phenytoin was associated with the deterioration, but so was the number of times that people had head injuries. That immediately suggests the possibility of fronto-temporal damage, but particularly frontal damage.

Dr S. W. Brown: We did try to exclude the ones with head injuries from our study and we might look at those separately.

General Discussion

Dr J. Duncan (Oxford): An interesting point that emerged from discussion with Dr Binnie was that by giving anti-epileptic drugs, TCI appeared to be reduced or abolished even though the spikes were still there.

Dr C.D. Binnie: Yes, the whole issue of treatment is a very difficult one. There are, at an anecdotal level, individual patients who clearly suffer disabilities due to TCI and who benefit from treatment. One phenomenon I have seen in a few patients following the administration of drugs is a breakdown of the relationship of the discharges to the cognitive impairment. They still have their discharges, but they are no longer associated with TCI. In view of what one knows about the lack of correlation in general between interictal discharges on the EEG and seizure frequency, this comes perhaps as no surprise. One action of the drugs seems to be to uncouple the clinical phenomenon and the EEG discharges.

Dr E.H. Reynolds: And yet presumably you gave the drugs because you thought you would do something to the discharges. The hypothesis was that the discharges were in some way responsible for your impairments on testing?

Dr C.D. Binnie: We found that without suppressing the discharges we were just apparently uncoupling them from the 'clinical manifestations'.

Dr E.H. Reynolds: Does that cast doubt in your mind on the association between the discharges and the TCI?

Dr C.D. Binnie: In a way I find it reassuring because sometimes subclinical discharges are associated with subtle clinical changes, but on the other hand inter-ictal EEGs are of little value for monitoring the progress of epilepsy. The relationship between discharges and clinical manifestations, including cognitive ones, is a subtle one, which we do not understand. Some drugs seem to be able to uncouple it. Some drugs make your EEG worse, even though the epilepsy gets better, some drugs make your epilepsy and your EEG better together.

Dr F.M.C. Besag: The terms clinical and subclinical are ones we need to re-examine. I would make a plea that we examine our subjects much more carefully. We may discover that some of the events we have been discussing as being subclinical discharges are actually associated with clinical manifestations, some of which Dr Binnie has very clearly shown, and some of which might have to be shown by more subtle psychological testing. We then get into a grey area. Where do we draw the dividing-line? How carefully do we have to test the subject before we decide there is no clinical manifestation with this discharge? I am very often faced with an abnormal child who has an abnormal EEG but who is not necessarily having seizures. What should we do, not with the subjects who have clear episodes of spike and wave, but with those who have frequent spikes on their EEG. Some of these subjects are not suffering clinically at all from these discharges. Others are very abnormal and have these discharges. When I sit down with the parents of such a child and show them the EEG I tell them that my approach is a very naïve one. Here we have an abnormal child and an abnormal EEG, I do not know whether the two are linked, but let us try to get the EEG more normal and see whether the child becomes normal as a result. In my experience sometimes he does, and that has been a worthwhile exercise. If, by the use of anticonvulsants, you do not make the child better then you withdraw them.

Dr E.H. Reynolds: What I am not clear about is whether there is a clinical problem. Dr Binnie has shown that in patients who are not complaining overtly of problems, he can detect cognitive impairment on testing which he relates to electrical discharges on the EEG. What will happen to these patients if we do not treat these discharges? What is the evidence that they are harmful?

Dr A.L. Rugland (Sandvika): I developed a test battery especially to assess subclinical discharges. We have many children and adults who have learning problems, even when their clinical seizures are well controlled. Many of them have subclinical discharges and the tests show that in many children with learning problems there is close connection between the discharges and their performance. I have some experience of treatment in these children, and have shown, up to now, a close connection between better performance and reduced frequency of subclinical discharges. I also have had a small number of children with no history of clinical seizures coming to me because they are doing poorly at school with subclinical discharges. We have had some good results using sodium valproate. However we have to monitor the dose carefully because we could lose what we have gained by taking away the discharge if we increase the dose too high.

Dr E.H. Reynolds: These are not epileptic children?

Dr A.L. Rugland: Most children whom I see have a history of epilepsy. However there is a small number that do not.

Professor N. O'Donohoe (Dublin): I think the condition of benign partial epilepsy or rolandic epilepsy has a key position here because it is recognized now to be the commonest single epileptic syndrome of childhood, and it is often associated with EEG discharges which may precede the onset of the syndrome by years. I have several patients who had abnormal EEGs years before they got their nocturnal seizures. Also the EEG abnormality lasts many years into adolescence, long after the epilepsy has ceased to be a problem. Now one of the features of these children is that they seem to be normal in other respects, and the condition is self limiting with a 100% recovery rate. We are not going to treat these children unless their seizures are frequent or upsetting. Certainly I would take issue with using a potentially dangerous drug like sodium valproate for conditions like this, and I prefer carbamazepine. Finally there is the Landau-Kleffner syndrome where children have a specific deficit, namely their inability to comprehend spoken language, usually with a very well defined EEG discharge and often with no epilepsy. Here the neurons seem incapable of normal function because they are discharging.

Dr E.H. Reynolds: At the moment you would not want to treat your patients with benign rolandic epilepsy with anticonvulsants?

Professor N. O'Donohoe: Not unless there was a clinical indication, and then only with carbamazepine.

Dr D.B. Smith: With regards to the apparent uncoupling that is seen with treatment of patients with TCI, this really reflects the inadequacy of the scalp-recorded EEG. We have had the opportunity to record several candidates for epilepsy surgery for one to two weeks with depth electrodes. During this time we frequently withdraw some or all of their medications in order to precipitate seizures. In several patients there is a dissociation between depth recorded seizures and scalp recorded seizures. Some have what we have been calling subclinical seizures, with brief lapses on video tape, which are really not apparent unless they are being interviewed or are attending to some test. These are accompanied by depth ictal discharges that may or may not be apparent on the surface. So one explanation for the uncoupling may be that as you treat, some of the depth ictal discharges are disappearing, but you are still seeing some of the scalp discharges from perhaps the lateral surface which may or may not be contributing to the clinical dysfunction. I think mesial temporal discharges are more associated with the clinical impairment than some of the more lateral discharges.

Dr M. Harper (Cardiff): There is a dangerous slippery slope here which we have to face. I would like to formulate a very dogmatic axiom. Just as we should not treat the EEG, so we should not treat subclinical abnormalities found on psychological or attention testing. That does of course raise the question of what is subclinical, and we may well have to define clinical in a rather more broad context. Unless we make some sort of dogmatic assertion vast numbers of children with all sorts of non-specific disorders are going to be exposed to the dangers of anticonvulsant medication.

Dr E.H. Reynolds: I quite agree with you. This is already beginning to happen as we have heard.

Dr M.R. Trimble: If a child has no overt motor seizure, is complaining of difficulties in the classroom, is referred to Dr Binnie or Dr Rugland who shows that there are discharges on the EEG which are related to performance on psychological tests, does that child have epilepsy? If the child has epilepsy, should you treat that child?

Professor J.A. Corbett: I think Dr Trimble is confusing the issue. Dr Harper has made a very clear statement which I think has a lot of merit in it. When Dr Trimble asks what do you do about this child, he refers to a child with classroom difficulties. This is a clinical problem. You do not have to ask has or has not this child got epilepsy? Let's forget that question. You are treating a clinical problem in a child with an EEG abnormality and you are treating the clinical problem with an anticonvulsant. You are not jumping to the conclusion that this child has epilepsy.

Dr M.R. Trimble: I was really chasing Dr Reynolds' definition of epilepsy.

Dr E.H. Reynolds: I agree with Dr Harper that epilepsy is a clinical diagnosis. I also sympathize with Professor Corbett's view but unfortunately people will continue to ask the question, and we will be forced to answer the question has this child got epilepsy? You may say it does not matter what you call it, and in a way you are right. But for a number of reasons, parents want to know, is it 'epilepsy'? What are the implications? Should it be treated with anti-epileptic drugs? It is quite clear that in this instance we are uncertain ourselves and, as far as possible, the word 'epilepsy' should be avoided. But the child with learning problems that we heard about did not have clinical epilepsy. Children are being treated with anti-epileptic drugs because something has been shown on the EEG.

Dr D.B. Smith: It is a very important issue if the child has a learning problem and every five minutes is having spike and wave discharges that last for three to four seconds, and the teacher and parents notice periods of inattention.

Dr M.R. Trimble: But these children did not even have that. They merely had an educational difficulty.

Dr C.D. Binnie: There are two questions that need to be addressed, and they are inseparable. The first one is, does this laboratory phenomenon of TCI lead to disabilities in psycho-social function? The second is, if such disabilities do exist are there any therapeutic measures which can be adopted to ameliorate them? I do not think you can reliably address the first without answering the second. We see children with spikes in their EEGs who have disabilities, but then there are many people with epilepsy who have disabilities. We see people with spikes without any disabilities but then the educational expectations of children with epilepsy are rather low. Perhaps they too could function better without their spikes. The only way to find out clearly whether this phenomenon is adversely affecting their pyscho-social function is to do what Dr Rugland is doing and attempt therapy, preferably in a properly controlled way because interventions affect teachers' expectations, to see whether there is an improvement. If there is, it is good evidence that the discharges are responsible for disabilities.

Professor N. O'Donohoe: I would like to quote two people. First, the great William Lennox who said that 'Epilepsy is a disease of the brain of which seizures are a symptom', and David Taylor who divided epilepsy into 'the disease, the illness and the predicaments'. The disease being the disease of the brain, the illness being the seizures and the predicaments being the associated problems. We have spent the last two days discussing predicaments. I would be inclined to support Dr Trimble in this way; it is as justifiable to treat the predicaments as it is to treat the illness or disease. If Dr Binnie's work is shown to be correct, then it is acceptable for us to use treatment for predicaments if we think it is going to help our patients.

Dr E.H. Reynolds: Can I slightly widen this discussion and bring in Dr Fenwick, whose talk emphasized the subject of depth recordings. Dr Smith said perhaps the drugs were suppressing something in the depths of the brain, but not on the surface. I found that a little difficult to understand, because what we see on the surface often begins in the depths. Yesterday, we had a very interesting talk from Dr Fenwick showing how different types of seizure arise from different areas of the brain, as revealed from depth electrode studies. Would you like to comment, Dr Fenwick, on the point that Dr Smith raised? Also, is it true, as I read in Penfield's work, that if you electrically stimulate the normal brain, for example the temporal lobe, you do not necessarily see the same phenomena that are observed in epileptic patients. He talks about 'epileptic sensitization' of the cortex. What is 'epileptic sensitization'? I also had the impression that phenomena are not quite so localized as we sometimes think by looking at diagrams derived from his studies; he could displace responses to electrical stimulation to different areas of the cortex. For example occasionally he could obtain a motor response from the sensory cortex, or a sensory response from the motor cortex. It is a very dynamic process that is going on.

Dr P.B.C. Fenwick: The important points I would like to draw out of that are the following: first, that with depth electrode studies we have to accept that what goes on in the depths and what goes on at the scalp are quite different. If we use a scalp EEG classification of epilepsy we may not be saying anything which is very intelligible. A generalized seizure may well start in the depths, in different parts of the depth. Therefore the track it takes and the structures which are involved at the onset of the seizure are quite different. Secondly, with regards to stimulation studies, there are several concepts which are involved. One is that stimulation of one area can produce different effects on different occasions. I do no think there is any doubt about that. The next one is that a lot of stimulation studies are done on abnormal brains which are already saturated with medication, and extrapolating to normal brains is a difficult process. The other point is that when you insert depth electrodes, you have no idea what disturbance they are causing to the wave forms that you measure. The best you can say is that these are arising from points of entry in an abnormal brain. The actual relationship between that and normal activity is very varied. What emerges is that there is great flexibility, but that there are patterns. Finally, there is a lot of difference between stimulation of the brain and seizure spread. To give you an example, Gloor says he never sees aggression arising from stimulation, but he does see aggression from seizures arising in a similar area to the stimulation site spreading throughout related structures. So stimulation studies and seizure spread are probably different.

Dr E.H. Reynolds: Are you worried therefore about this concept of treating surface electrical discharges in children who perhaps do not have epilepsy?

Dr P.B.C. Fenwick: We are talking about things at different levels. Obviously, if you are a clinician and a child presents to you with a clinical disorder, then you may give anticonvulsants. If I can take it into my field, if you have adults with paroxysmal disorders of behaviour, e.g. aggressive disorders, which you think are possibly epileptic, you are perfectly permitted to try these people on anticonvulsants. But I think that is different from the research aspect where you are looking at the relationship between these discharges and behaviour.

Dr M.R. Trimble: Dr Fenwick, what is the relationship of the amygdala and hippo-campus to the genesis of hallucinations and illusions?

Dr P.B.C. Fenwick: The argument is that these structures are involved with hallucinations and illusions. In the stimulation studies one can ask how far did the stimulation spread by looking at after discharges. The interesting thing is that the phenomena are usually associated with after discharges. If this is the case then you have got quite widespread changes and these may influence particular trigger areas. But in some of the work there are no after discharges. That is much more difficult to explain, because then one is looking at very specific limitations to the structures involved. The only way that you can argue from there is that you are tapping specific pathways which are involved in the process of hallucinations.

Dr M.R. Trimble: The after discharges are usually confined to the limbic system?

Dr P.B.C. Fenwick: Yes, although sometimes they do spread into the nearby cortex. The point about these studies is that they can occur without after discharges.

Dr M.R. Trimble: Why did Penfield find so few people that had experiential phenomena from cortical stimulation?

Dr P.B.C. Fenwick: I do not know. There are part answers to it. There are obviously very specific cortical areas where you get responses every time, for example in the primary receiving cortex. There are areas of the cortex which are very specific, there are other areas where you might expect to get changes but do not. I expect this is something to do with primary spread.

Professor J.A. Corbett: I would like to add another word about the nomenclature of cognitive deteroration and dementia in epilepsy. Some people will be familiar with the proposed classification for ICD 10. I think it represents a major advance. The main improvements are in the classification of developmental disorders and particularly specific disorders. I cannot go along with this concept of an epileptic dementia. The late Professor Pond stated that in most cases, when severe deterioration is seen, the problem usually starts in childhood, although it may come on later in adolescence or adult life. I am quite happy to describe that as dementia in people with epilepsy, but not as 'epileptic dementia', which implies that it is a syndrome. Dementia in people with epilepsy implies that you still keep your options open between a number of different pathologies.

As far as children are concerned, I would not use the term dementia because, as we have heard, there is uncertainty whether there is arrest in some cases or deterioration in others. I would like to stick to the terms deterioration and arrest as being useful concepts. We have found when we have looked very carefully at cases, that we can probably make a diagnosis in eight out of ten. Some of them clearly fit into the Lennox–Gastaut syndrome, the occasional one has infantile spasms and deterioration. They particularly show pervasive disintegrative disorders, with marked impairments in social interaction and language. We find others who seem to have had some acute phenytoin encephalopathy, which may improve when you change their medication. Others have other conditions. Maybe a very small proportion of cases in both adults and children will emerge with a dementia of epilepsy, but at the moment I think we should regard these as a small group of cases, aetiology unknown.

Dr S.W. Brown: I am not proposing that there is an epileptic dementia. I was suggesting that some of those patients whose intellectual deterioration cannot be explained by other means are displaying a type of severe frontal lobe syndrome, which might be confused with dementia.

Dr M.R. Trimble: Dr Reynolds is keen on the Gowers' phenomenon; one seizure begets the next. We have heard that the temporal lobes are intimately linked with a number of important psychological functions, particularly memory. If you have a process going on in the temporal lobes, and we know now that it may involve endogenous neurotoxins which themselves destroy neurons, must we not keep alive the concept of a progressive epileptic dementia which is specifically interlinked with the epileptic process. This may become more progressive as limbic system after discharges affect other areas of the brain?

Professor J.A. Corbett: Yes, I am prepared to believe that it exists, but it accounts for a minority of people who have been described as having epileptic deterioration. I think we should study this group very carefully to see whether they have frontal lobe syndromes or, as I suspect and have seen, very severe memory deficits.

Dr M.R. Trimble: Dr Reynolds suggests that this a very common phenomenon in epilepsy, that one seizure begets the next, that there is a process of neuronal change going on within the brain.

Dr E.H. Reynolds: I have not said anything about dementia or other psychological aspects. I have only been talking about the control of seizures. My observations are that we can control 75% of newly diagnosed epileptic patients which contrasts with the difficulty we have in controlling chronic patients. We asked the question how do newly diagnosed patients become chronic patients? The conventional answer is that they have more severe epilepsy from the start. That, however, is a very difficult concept and an alternative way of looking at it is that epileptic patients become more and more chronic as was proposed by Gowers 100 years ago. I shall not enlarge upon Gowers' hypothesis any further but our own observations are in keeping with that idea. Dr Trimble is extrapolating from that to similar sorts of concepts for psychological dysfunction; I agree that this is quite possible.

Dr M.R. Trimble: That chronic group is also identified by more severe neuro-psychological and neuropsychiatric deficits.

Dr E.H. Reynolds: Yet, but these patients have more frequent seizures, they have more drugs and more psychological and social complications and so it becomes very complicated.

Professor J.A. Corbett: Professor O'Donohoe, the Lennox–Gastaut syndrome seems to be increasingly emerging as an entity, although there is a question that it is West's syndrome occurring at a later age. Do you think this phenomenon of failure to control seizures accounts for the intellectual deterioration you see in the Lennox-Gastaut syndrome?

Professor N. O'Donohoe: There was a meeting in Germany last September specifically on the Lennox–Gastaut syndrome. They tried to define the syndrome very specifically as a condition which arises de novo rather than a condition which arises in previously handicapped children. Some other criteria are that these children show mental arrest and/or deterioration and they show specific EEG patterns. Everyone's experience of Lennox–Gastaut syndrome is that it is remarkably resistant to our present methods of treatment, including dietetic treatment. The question of whether frequent seizures cause deterioration is unanswerable. It has been speculated that the Lennox–Gastaut syndrome is primarily an encephalopathy of some kind, but the aetiology is unknown except that it can be triggered off by a multiplicity of events.

Dr Harper: Is the Gowers phenomenon due to the epilepsy or is it the underlying condition? Careful neuropathological studies on patients who have had many ECTs who have not shown any spontaneous fits or any deterioration of cognitive dysfunction, suggests it is more the underlying condition that generates the epilepsy which leads to the unresponsive case, rather than the occurrence of seizures.

Dr E.H. Reynolds: The Gowers' phenomenon requires investigation. The implication is that you should treat early and prevent evolving problems. Obviously the observations about ECT are very relevant but I did not realize it was as cut and dried as you actually implied. My last comment concerns this issue of early versus delayed treatment. A recent study in the *British Journal of Psychiatry* on the treatment in schizophrenia indicated that if you delay treatment the outlook is rather worse than if you give early treatment. This may be true for many neuro-psychiatric conditions.

Index

absence seizures, *see* petit mal epilepsy
age, relationship to neuropsychological
    measures 70–2, 74–5
age of onset
  behaviour disorders and 104
  cognitive function and 101
  deterioration of IQ and 117–18
  memory impairment and 167
  see also late onset epilepsy
aggressive behaviour 36–8
  subcortical EEG discharges associated
    with 52, 53
AIDS 90
alcoholism
  dementia in 195
  seizures in 191, 193–5, 199
Alzheimer's disease 116, 190, 193, 200
amino acids, neurotoxic (excitotoxins)
    130, 166, 206
amygdala, EEG discharges in 52, 54, 58,
    205–6
anti-epileptic drugs, *see* anticonvulsant
    drugs
anticonvulsant drugs (AEDs)
  in alcoholics 199
  attention and concentration and 21
  behavioural effects 67–77, 105, 138–41,
    159–160
  in children 93–4, 102, 105, 120–1, 138
  cognitive deterioration and 120–1, 179–
    180, 181
  cognitive effects 67–77, 82–3, 102, 121,
    135–8, 141
  effects on mood 139–41, 150–1, 161
  memory impairment and 17–18, 136,
    168, 171
  mental speed and 18–19, 136
  monitoring serum levels 35
  in 'subclinical' epilepsy 48–9, 202, 203–4

transitory cognitive impairment (TCI)
    and 201
  see also polytherapy
antidepressants 151
anxiety 152
  effects of anticonvulsant drugs (AEDs)
    on 140
Aretaeus 113
arteriosclerosis 192
aryl sulphatase A deficiency, partial 116
attention
  assessment of 19–21, 22
  memory impairment and 172–3
Attentional Battery 172
auras, temporal lobe 58, 60
automatisms
  frontal lobe 62–3
  temporal lobe 59, 60

Batten's disease 116, 131
Bear-Fedio inventory 30, 140, 147
Beck Depression Inventory 30
behaviour
  anticonvulsant drug effects 67–77, 105,
    138–41, 159–160
  effects of fronto-temporal dysfunction
    on 187
  in prodrome 161
behaviour disorders 27–38
  aggressive behaviour 36–8
  assessment methods 29–35
    direct observation 33–4
    interviews 29–30
    neuropsychological assessment 34–5
    questionnaires 30–2
    reliability and validity 31
    self-monitoring 32–3
  in children
    cognitive function and 106

208

behaviour disorders, in children
  (*contd.*)
    factors affecting 103–6, 139
    prevalence 103
  definitions 27–8
  paroxysmal, EEG discharges and 51–
    64, 79–80, 81–2
  types 28, 29
benign partial epilepsy (rolandic epilepsy)
    61, 81, 90, 202–3
Benton Visual Retention Test 14
benzodiazepines, memory impairment
    and 166; *see also* clobazam *and*
    clonazepam
Binswanger's disease 192
brain abscess 196
brain damage
  behaviour disorders in 103–4
  during seizures 121
  epilepsy caused by 116
  memory impairment and 166
  see also head injury *and* organic
    (symptomatic) epilepsy
Bristol Social Adjustment Score 92

Caesar, Julius 13, 145, 146
carbamazepine (CBZ) 93
  behavioural effects 67–9, 73–7, 105,
    139, 140, 141, 159
  cognitive deterioration and 121
  cognitive effects 67–9, 73–7, 102, 136–7,
    138
  memory function and 17, 168
  mental speed and 18–19
  psychotropic effects 139, 141, 150
cerebral infections 116, 191, 196
cerebral trauma, *see* head injury
cerebral tumours 93, 191, 195–6
cerebrovascular disorders 190–1, 192–3
childhood epilepsy
  behaviour disorders in 103–6, 139
  benign partial (rolandic) 61, 81, 90,
    202–3
  cognitive deterioration in 11, 113–24
    causes 115–16
    concept of developmental arrest 122–
      4, 129, 130–1
    evidence for 114–15
    factors affecting 117–21
  cognitive function 97–102, 138
  data sources 87–8
  educational needs 87–95

improving medical services 95
intellectual ability (IQ) 10, 97–8
investigations 92–3
management 93–4
possible causes 89–90
prevalence 88–9
social factors 90–1
'subclinical' 202, 203, 204
see also educational performance *and*
  schools
clobazam
  behaviour disorders and 105
  cognitive effects 19, 136, 137
clonazepam
  in children 93–4
  cognitive effects 136, 141
cognitive function
  anticonvulsant drug effects 67–77, 82–3,
    102, 121, 135–8, 141
  assessment of 9–22, 69–70
  behaviour disorders and 34–5, 106
  in children 97–102
  deterioration in
    in children 113–24
    cortical localization 184–6
    nature and extent of 182, 183–4
    see also dementia
  factors affecting 99–102
  transitory impairment, *see* transitory
    cognitive impairment (TCI)
  variable impairment 121–2
  see also attention; educational
    performance; intelligence;
    learning problems; memory
    disorders *and* mental speed
cognitive task analysis 22
complex partial seizures
  depression and 147–8
  frontal lobe 62–3
  temporal lobe 58
computer assisted tomography (CT scans)
  92–3
computer monitor screens 90
computer television games 46
concentration 19–21, 22
confusion, post-ictal 122
Continuous Performance Test (CPT) 20
Creutzfeld-Jakob disease 193–4
CT scans 92–3

dementia 131, 177–87, 200, 206–7
  aetiology 190–6

cortical locus of cognitive impairment in
    184–6
evidence for 178–84
prevalence 189–190
primary alcoholic 195
see also cognitive function,
    deterioration in and intelligence
depression 145–151, 152
    anticonvulsant drugs (AEDs) and
        140–1, 161
    interictal 146–150
    peri-ictal 146
    seizure frequency and 148, 161
    suicide and parasuicide 150
    treatment 150–1
depth recorded seizures 56, 82, 203, 204–6
    behavioural effects 52–6, 79–80
    in frontal lobe epilepsy 61–4
    in temporal lobe epilepsy (TLE) 56–61
developmental arrest 123–4, 129, 130–1
diaries, for monitoring problem
        behaviours 32–3
diphenylhydantoin, see phenytoin
dorso-lateral frontal seizures 62
DPH, see phenytoin
driving motor vehicles, subclinical EEG
        discharges and 48
drug-induced seizures 191
duration of epilepsy
    behaviour disorders and 104
    cognitive deterioration and 118–19
    memory impairment and 167

ECT (electroconvulsive therapy) 161, 207
education 87
    memory impairment and 169
    in normal schools 91–2
    relationship to behavioural measures
        70–2, 74–5
    special 88, 91, 94–5, 131–2
    see also schools
educational performance 91, 98–9, 115
    behaviour disorders and 106
    factors affecting 99–102
    subclinical EEG discharges and 48, 202,
        203–4
EEG 35, 92
EEG discharges
    behaviour disorders and 51–64, 104–5
    cognitive function and 18, 45–9, 101–2
    in primary cerebral degenerative
        disorders 193, 194

subclinical, see subclinical EEG
        discharges
subcortical 52–64, 79–80, 81–2, 203,
        204–6
elation 150
elderly
    dementia in 189–190
    epilepsy in 190
    see also late onset epilepsy
employment prospects 95
encephalitis, epilepsy and dementia
        caused by 196
environment
    effects on behaviour disorders 105–6
    effects on cognitive function 102
epilepsy
    age of onset, see age of onset
    in childhood, see childhood epilepsy
    definitions of 82, 202–3
    duration of, see duration of epilepsy
    historical aspects 3–7
    idiopathic, cognitive function in 99–
        100, 117
    'larval' 5, 45
    organic, see organic (symptomatic)
        epilepsy
    subclinical, see subclinical EEG
        discharges
epilepsy partialis continuans 61
ethosuximide 93, 102

family
    assessment of behaviour disorders 29–
        30, 34
    communication with schools 94, 129–30
    effects on behaviour disorders 105–6
    effects on cognitive function 102
    one-parent, childhood epilepsy
        and 90–1
flicker-associated seizures 90
folic acid deficiency 159–160
Fragile X syndrome 90
frequency of seizures, see seizure
        frequency
frontal lobe dysfunction in dementia 187
frontal lobe seizures, depth electrode
        studies 61–4
fugue states, post-ictal 122

generalized seizures
    cognitive function and 15, 119–20
    frontal lobe 63

generalized seizures (*contd.*)
  primary 80–1
Gowers, William R. 4, 5, 113–14
Gowers' phenomenon 206, 207–8

hallucinations, genesis of 53–6, 58, 205
Halstead-Reitan Neuropsychological Test
    Battery 69
Hamilton Depression Rating Scale
    (HDRS) 148–9
head injury 116, 196, 199, 200
  during seizures 121
  memory and attention and 173
hepatocerebral degeneration in
    alcoholism 195
herpes simplex encephalitis 196
hippocampus, EEG discharges in 52, 54,
    58, 205–6
Hippocrates 3–4, 145
Hospital Anxiety and Depression (HAD)
    scale 30
Huntington's disease 193
hypomania 151–2

idiopathic (non-organic) epilepsy,
    cognitive function in 99–100, 117
illusions, genesis of 58, 205
infantile spasms (West syndrome) 119,
    124, 206, 207
infections, central nervous system 116,
    191, 196
intellectual ability, *see* intelligence (IQ)
intelligence (IQ)
  behaviour disorders and 106
  deterioration in 11–12, 114–15
    causes 115–16
    concept of developmental arrest 122–
        4, 129, 130–1
    factors affecting 117–21
    see also dementia
  factors affecting 99–102
  levels 10–11, 70, 76, 97–8
  relationship to age and education 70–2,
      74–5
intelligence (IQ) tests 10–13, 21, 178, 182
  lateralization of lesions and 12, 13
  uses 12–13
interviews, for assessment of behaviour
    disorders 29–30
intracranial haemorrhages 196

Jackson, Hughlings 5–6

Lafayette Repeatable
    Neuropsychological Battery 69
Landau-Kleffner syndrome 90, 202
'larval' epilepsy 5, 45
late onset epilepsy 189–96, 200
  aetiology 190–6
  epidemiology 189–190
lateralization of lesions
  cognitive function and 12, 13, 46–7
  depressive illness and 148–50, 152
  memory impairment and 15–16, 167–8,
      171
learning problems 13–18, 98–9
  memory impairment and 169, 171
  methods of assessment 14–15
  subclinical discharges and 202, 204
  see also educational performance *and*
      memory
Lennox-Gastaut syndrome 119, 124, 206,
    207
lie scoring 32
limbic system, abnormal discharges from
    52–6, 82, 205–6

magneto-encephalography 56, 64
mania 151–2
Marchiafava-Bignami disease 195
medical records 35
memory disorders 13–18, 165–73, 199
  anticonvulsant drugs and 17–18, 136,
      168, 171
  attention and 172–3
  in children 99, 101
  factors influencing 15–18, 166–8
  methods of assessment 14–15, 21–2, 169
  nature of 168–73
  in right versus left temporal lobe
      epilepsy (TLE) 15–16, 167–8, 171
  subictal EEG discharges and 16–17, 166
  type of seizures and 15, 167–8
Memory Quotient (MQ) 14, 169
meningiomas 200
meningitis
  bacterial 196
  tuberculous 196
mental age, arrested development
    of 123–4, 129, 130–1
mental speed (psychomotor function)
    18–19, 99, 136
Minnesota Multiphasic Personality
    Inventory (MMPI) 30, 139, 146–7

mood
  effects of anticonvulsant drugs
    on 139–41, 150–1
  epilepsy and 145–52
  memory impairment and 168
  see also depression
Mood Adjective Check List 140
motor area, supplementary, seizures in
  61–2
motor cortex, focal status of 61
motor seizures, major, cognitive function
  and 119
motor speed, effects of anticonvulsant
  drugs on 19, 136
motor vehicles, driving, subclinical EEG
  discharges and 48
myoclonus in Creutzfeldt-Jakob disease
  193–4

National Childhood Development Study
  (NCDS) 88
neurodegenerative diseases 116, 190, 191,
  192–4
neurology, relationship to psychiatry 5–7
neuropsychological assessment 9–22,
  34–5, 47–8, 69–70
neurotoxins (excitotoxins) 130, 166, 206

observation of problem behaviours 33–4
opercular seizures 60
orbital frontal seizures 62
organic (symptomatic) epilepsy
  behaviour disorders in 103–4
  cognitive function in 99–100, 117
  see also brain damage

panencephalitis, subacute sclerosing 116
parasuicide 150
parents, communication with schools
  94–5, 129–30
pattern-associated seizures 90
pellagratous cerebral damage in
  alcoholism 195
perceptuomotor performance 19, 136–7
personality disturbances 6, 187
petit mal epilepsy (absence seizures) 89
  cognitive function and 100, 119, 124
phenobarbitone (phenobarbital, Pb) 93,
  160
  behavioural effects 67–9, 73–7, 105
  cognitive effects 67–9, 73–7, 102, 137
  effects on mood 139, 140, 141, 150

memory function and 17, 168
polytherapy 137–8
phenytoin (DPH, PHT) 93, 159
  behavioural effects 67–9, 73–7, 105,
    139, 140
  cognitive deterioration and 120–1, 123,
    124, 200
  cognitive effects 67–9, 73–7, 102, 136–7,
    141
  memory function and 17, 18, 136, 168
  mental speed and 18–19, 136
  polytherapy 137–8
Pick's disease 193
polytherapy 67
  cognitive effects 17–18, 21, 102, 137–8
  effects on mood 140–1
posterior temporal neo-cortical seizures
  60
primidone (PRM)
  behavioural and cognitive effects 67–9,
    73–7, 102, 168
  in children 93, 102, 160
  effects on mood 139
prodrome
  behavioural changes 161
  variable cognitive impairment in 121–2
Profile of Mood Scales (POMS) 70
'pseudodepressed syndrome' 187
'pseudopsychopathic syndrome' 187
psychiatric illness, history of epilepsy as
  4–7
psychomotor seizures, see temporal lobe
  epilepsy (TLE)
psychomotor speed (mental speed) 18–19,
  99, 136
psychotherapy 150
psychotropic effects of carbamazepine
  139, 141

questionnaires for assessment of
  behaviour disorders 30–2

Reaction Times (RTs) 18, 19
records, medical and social 35
reliability of assessment methods 31, 33
Rett syndrome 90
Rey Auditory Verbal Learning Test
  (RAVLT) 14
rolandic epilepsy (benign partial epilepsy)
  61, 81, 90, 202–3
role play 33–4

schizophrenia
  epileptiform discharges in 53–6
  intellectual deterioration in 131
schizophreniform psychoses, postictal and
    interictal 122
scholastic performance, *see* educational
    performance
schools
  communication with 94–5, 129–30
  mainstream 91–2
  medical services at 95
  special 88, 91, 94–5, 129–30
  see also education
seizure frequency
  behaviour disorders and 104
  cognitive deterioration and 120, 178–9
  cognitive function and 101
  depression and 148, 161
  memory impairment and 166
seizure types
  behaviour disorders and 104
  cognitive deterioration and 119–20
  cognitive function and 100–1
  see also specific types of seizures
seizures
  depth recorded, *see* depth recorded
    seizures
  misconceptions about 29–30
  prodromal period, *see* prodrome
  self-monitoring 33
  variable cognitive impairment
    associated with 121–2
self-monitoring of behaviour problems
    32–3
septum, EEG discharges in 52, 54
sex
  behaviour disorders and 105
  cognitive function and 102
  intellectual deterioration and 184,
    186–7
Signoret's Memory Battery Scale 169
social adjustment of school-aged children
    92
social class, childhood epilepsy and 90–1
social records 35
social skills, assessment of 31–2
Spielberger Scales of anxiety 30
staff, assessment of behaviour disorders
    by 29, 30, 34
status, non-convulsive 122
status epilepticus, cognitive deterioration
    caused by 124, 130

Sternberg memory scanning task 14, 17,
  21
Stroop test 20–1, 172
subacute sclerosing panencephalitis 116
subclinical EEG discharges 5, 101–2
  memory impairment and 16–17, 166
  transitory cognitive impairment
    and 45–9, 201–2
  treatment 48–9, 202, 203–4
subdural haemorrhages 196
subictal EEG discharges, *see* subclinical
    EEG discharges
suicide 150
supplementary motor area seizures 61–2
symptomatic epilepsy, *see* organic
    epilepsy

TCI, *see* transitory cognitive impairment
tempero-basal limbic seizures 60
temporal lobe epilepsy (TLE)
  in children 89–90
  cognitive function in 119
  depression in 147–150
  depth electrode studies 56–61
  lateralization of lesions, *see*
    lateralization of lesions
  memory impairment in 15–16, 167–8,
    169, 171
  personality and behaviour in 6, 187
  suicide risks 150
temporal lobectomy, psychoses after 161
temporal polar seizures 60
transitory cognitive impairment
    (TCI) 45–9, 79, 80, 122, 204
  detection 46–7
  neuropsychological testing and 47–8
  practical implications 48–9
  treatment 48–9, 201
tuberculous meningitis 196
tuberose sclerosis 130

validity of assessment methods 31, 33
valproate, sodium 93
  behaviour disorders and 105
  cognitive deterioration and 121
  cognitive effects 19, 102, 136–7
  memory impairment and 168
vigilance 19–21, 22
viloxazine 151
visual scanning task 20, 21
visuomotor coordination 99, 101
visuoperceptual function 99

Washington Psychosocial Inventory
   (WPSI) 32
Wechsler intelligence scales (WAIS and
   WISC) 10–13, 21, 69–70
Wechsler Memory Scale (WMS) 14, 169
Wernicke-Korsakoff syndrome 195

West syndrome (hypsarrhythmia/infantile
   spasms) 119, 124, 206, 207
Wilson's disease 194

Zazzo test 172